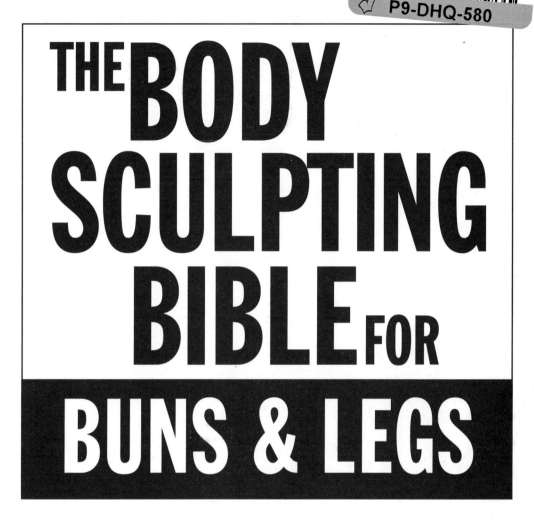

THE BODY SCULPTING BIBLE FOR BUNS & LEGS

James Villepigue
Hugo Rivera

Photography by
Peter Field Peck

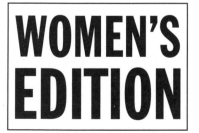

WOMEN'S EDITION

healthylivingbooks
New York • London

www.bodysculptingbible.com

A HEALTHY LIVING BOOK
Published by Hatherleigh Press
5-22 46th Avenue, Suite 200
Long Island City, NY 11101
www.healthylivingbooks.com

Villepigue, James C.
 The body sculpting bible for buns & legs: women's edition / by James Villepigue
    p. cm.
 ISBN 1-57826-213-5
 1. Bodybuilding for women. 2. Exercise for women. I. Title.
 GV546.6.W64V545 2004
 613.6'6082—dc22
                    2005021995

Seek the advice of your physician before starting any physical fitness program.

Healthy Living Books are available for bulk purchase, special promotions, and premiums. For information on reselling and special purchase opportunities, please call us at 1-800-528-2550 and ask for the Special Sales Manager.

Special thanks to our models, Rebecca Houck and Regina Cantoni-Hagen, and to RoseMarie Alfieri.

Cover and interior design by Deborah Miller.

10 9 8 7 6 5 4 3 2 1
Printed in Canada

Dedication

I would like to dedicate this exciting project to the most important people in my life. To my mom, Nancy, a genuine angel on Earth: I am truly blessed by God to be your son and I simply adore you. To my beautiful and talented sister, Debbie, aka Deborah: My love for you could never cease and I am, as I have always said, "So very proud of you!" To my awesome dad, Jim: I love you more than you could ever know. I miss you so much pal. Thank you for helping me to become the man I am...Warrior Overwhelmed...I love you, I adore you, and I honor you every moment of my life. God bless you, pal! To God, thank you, thank you, thank you! To my fiancée, Heather: Thank you again for all of your incredible and much needed support. I love you and look forward to our wonderful life together. To all of my beautiful family, loved ones, and friends: You all know who you are and I love you all very much!

Finally, to all of you reading, I owe a great debt of gratitude to you all. Thank you so very much for your interest in our work. We truly hope you enjoy. Believe and achieve. God bless!

James

Dedication

First of all, I would like to thank God for giving me the talent and the ability to not only be a writer, but also for allowing me to make a living doing what I love.

Having said that, I would like to dedicate this book to my number one fans and biggest supporters in the world, my lovely wife Lina and my son Chad. I could not be anywhere near where I am today if it would not be for your love and support Lina. From the bottom of my heart, thank you so much for everything you have ever done for me. Chad, by seeing how hard you work in school and how industrious you are, you inspire me to be even better every day; thanks so much pal.

I also want to dedicate this book to my parents Haydeé and Arturo, my grandparents Nydia and Dr. Raul Rivera, and my great grandmother María Mercedes in Puerto Rico, who have always supported me from the day I was born and who ensured that I always had what I needed in order to be successful. Also, for instilling in me the belief that if you put your mind to it you can accomplish anything. Also, to my brothers Raul and Javier Rivera for their support and encouragement. In addition, I want to dedicate this book to my in-laws Edith and Alvaro, who have always treated me as their own son and who have supported my endeavors in every way, shape or form possible.

I want to also give thanks to my co-author and great friend James Villepigue, for without his help, I could not be where I am today either. Jimmy, you are a great human being and an awesome friend. To my good friend William Kemp for all of his faith in me and superb advice. Bill, it is a true honor to know you and I thank you for all you have ever done for me. Always thanks to Dave and Laree Draper, for their help in introducing me to this great industry. To Stella Juarez, author of Stella's Kitchen, for her support, friendship, and for motivating me to apply to become the new www.bodybuilding.about.com guide. To Brian Ward who is one of the best friends anyone can have. Brian, I cannot thank you enough for all the support you have given me in these past few years. You're the man. To Peter Peck, who is the most talented and passionate photographer I have ever known. Without you, Peter, the books would only be half complete. To everyone at Hatherleigh, Andrew, Kevin, Andrea, Alyssa, Debbie, Erin, RoseMarie and everyone else that helps make these publications possible, a big thank you! And last but certainly not least, to my fans and avid readers who at the end of the day are the only reason that I exist. Thank you so much for all your support and please know that I am here to help you achieve all your fitness goals.

All the best!
Hugo

Table of Contents

Precautions

You should always consult a physician before starting any weight gain or fat reduction training/nutrition program.

A basic metabolic test, thyroid, lipid and testosterone panel is recommended prior to starting this program in order to detect anything that can prevent you from making the most out of your efforts.

Consult your doctor regarding these tests.

If you are unfamiliar with any of the exercises, consult an experienced trainer to instruct you on the proper form and execution of the unfamiliar exercise. Improper form can lead to injury.

The instructions and advice presented herein are not intended as a substitute for medical or other personal professional counseling.

Introduction
Is This Workout for You?

When we wrote the original *Body Sculpting Bible for Women,* our goal was to provide women with a comprehensive whole-body workout program based on proven methods of training that we've used with clients, who have achieved great results. The response to the book has been fabulous and we are grateful and gratified to all who have found the book helpful in their quest for a healthy, fit, sculpted body.

Readers also have shared their opinions about the book and offered suggestions for the future. This book is a result of your suggestions: namely that you are particularly concerned about slimming and toning your lower body. This is not surprising to us; if we were to poll our female clients regarding the body parts they would most like to slim, reshape or sculpt, the most common responses would be their butts, thighs, and waists. For most women, these are the areas

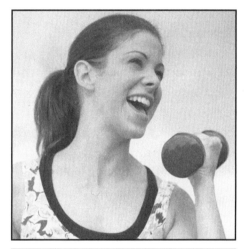

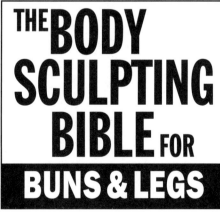

THE BODY SCULPTING BIBLE FOR BUNS & LEGS

where excess fat is stored—the jiggly parts—and which seem, despite—perhaps because of—severely restrictive diets, resistant to weight loss efforts. This can cause loss of motivation to exercise.

The thighs and butt are hot spots that are not easy to hide when you have excess fat. It's not easy being overweight, having to deal with our insecurity over how others perceive us and the way we look. It would be nice if we really didn't care how we looked or what others thought. Unfortunately, the reality is that we often look to others for approval in the hope that they look at us and see us as beautiful people. Whether for our loved ones or strangers on the street, why wouldn't we want to look awesome? When we look awesome, we feel awesome and the benefits go on and on. Think about that glorious day in the near future when you will finally rid your closet of the overly loose garments and drapery you've been wearing for so long. Think about the wonderful rewards you will give yourself, once you've achieved those beautifully sculpted legs and butt. Once you achieve your personal fitness goals, you can't imagine how amazingly different and great you will feel.

In the past, women believed they could spot reduce to achieve slimmer, toned legs and butts. And so we would see women at the gym doing a hundred leg lifts to rid themselves of the dimples in their outer thighs. Unfortunately, this technique does not work, and despite the evidence for this we continue to see people who perform redundant exercises and endless and wasteful repetitions, in the belief that it is helping to tone muscles and shave fat.

As we now all know, the only way to lose actual fat in your body—regardless of where it is stored—is to eat a healthy, calorie-appropriate diet, engage in cardiovascular exercise to burn the actual fat, and perform resistance or weight training with the proper weight and number of reps and sets, to sculpt, and add beautiful definition, and to increase your body's basal metabolic rate.

The Body Sculpting Bible for Buns and Legs presents a full-body weight-training program that focuses on your lower body, to home in on your butt and legs so that you can reveal latent muscular definition, giving you a look that is fit, shapely, strong, and feminine. Done in conjunction with a full-body workout (such as in *The Body Sculpting Bible*) that includes cardiovascular sessions, and while following a healthy diet, these workouts will reshape your legs and butt—improving the way you look in everything you wear, whether in a party outfit or bikini. Sound good?

In Part One of the book we discuss the anatomy and exercise science for the lower body, so that you can understand how these muscles are meant to function and how to select the appropriate exercise for each muscle group. We also reveal the makeup of the program, which offers three levels of workouts: beginner, intermediate, and advanced. While many of the exercises involve using free weights for resistance, there are also machine options to ensure that your workouts are varied.

Chapter Two provides a discussion of our recommended balanced approach to nutrition in which we offer nutritional guidelines to make choosing the most nutritious, calorie appropriate foods easier.

Part Two of the book contains detailed descriptions of the exercises you will find in your workout for the major muscles of the lower body—the quads and glutes, hamstrings, calves, outer and inner thigh muscles, and abdominals—and includes a chapter on lower body stretches for your post-workout stretch.

In Part Three you'll find the three programs, which are based on the training principle of periodization in which you vary your routine every couple of weeks in order to continually surprise and challenge your muscles. You can use these programs as stand-alone workouts in conjunction with upper body routines of your choice, or incorporate them into the full body workout programs of the original *Body Sculpting Bible.* It's up to you.

With the Buns & Legs Workouts you can expect to sculpt the leaner legs, that better butt, and those awesome abs you've always wanted. Welcome to a new lower body!

Part I
A Sexy Lower Body

To sculpt your glutes and quads into perfect shape you need to have some understanding of the muscles of the lower body and how they function. This chapter goes into some basics in anatomy and kinesiology (a study of body movements), before discussing the specifics of your Buns & Legs Workout protocol.

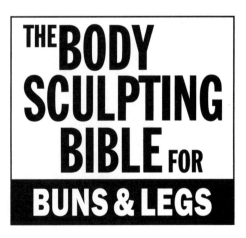

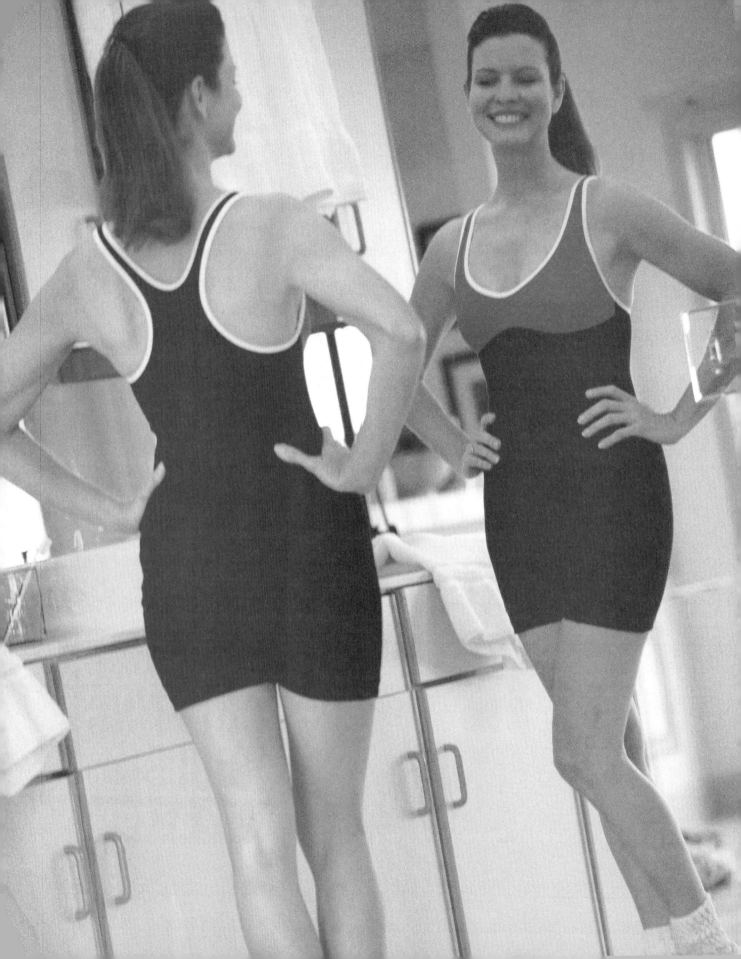

Chapter 1

Sculpting Your Best Butt and Leaner Legs

The Buns & Legs Workout homes in on the major muscles of your lower body to give you sleek and sexy legs and a shapely firm butt. In particular, it works the gluteus maximus, medius, and minimus muscles, (the muscles that define and shape your buttocks); the biceps femoris (hamstrings) at the backs of your legs; the rectus femoris (quadriceps) muscles in the fronts of your thighs; the tensor fasciae latae (muscles at the sides of your thighs also know as the hip abductors); the adductor muscles of the inner thigh, and the gastrocenemius and soleus muscles in your calves.

When you work the larger muscle groups of the buttocks and quadriceps, you also work the

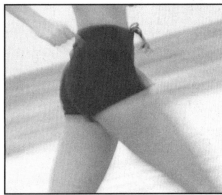

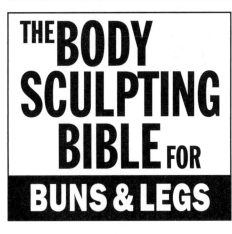

THE BODY SCULPTING BIBLE FOR BUNS & LEGS

1

smaller muscles of the lower body. For example, when performing a leg press, you are not only working your larger gluteal muscles but also are training your hamstrings, which act as secondary helper or assisting muscles. For this reason, it is generally recommended to work the larger muscle groups first in a given workout session. Otherwise, you will tire the helper muscles out and they will not be able to work as effectively when you perform your squat or lunge. There are times, however, when you may want to work out the smaller muscles first—on those days when your primary focus is on the hamstrings, say, or the inner thigh.

When you work your leg muscles, you will be able to use weight that is much heavier than when you train the muscles in your upper body. Your legs are the powerhouse muscles in your body and they are already quite strong because you use them every day just walking around, climbing stairs, and in most of the activities of your daily life.

EXERCISES FOR A SLEEK LOWER BODY

Let's take a look at how the muscles of your lower body function: The gluteus maximus muscles act at the hip joint and are responsible for extending your hip and also for rotating your hip laterally. In order to train the gluteals you need to use resistance to perform hip extension and rotation. Exercises such as the squat and leg press are terrific here. The primary function of the gluteus medius and minimus is to abduct your hip (or move your leg away from the midline of your body). Training these muscles involves performing movements in which you press your leg out to the side and rotate it. Your hamstrings run from behind your knees to your hips and their primary function also is hip extension and knee flexion. Good exercises include hamstring curls and stiff-legged dead lifts. The quadriceps, at the fronts of your legs, are opposing muscles to the hamstrings—in other words, they perform the opposite function. Where the hamstrings extend your hips and flex your knees, the quadriceps flex your hips and extends your knee. Classic quadriceps exercises are the knee extension and modified lunge. To work your calf muscles, which act at your ankle and foot, you need to perform plantar flexion (pressing your toes into the floor while lifting the heels).

A wide variety of exercises target the lower body muscles. Taking advantage of this variety is one of the keys to success in achieving great legs and buns. It's easy to get into an exercise rut; to continue to do the same exercises for muscle groups in the same ways, without variation. The problem with this approach is that you are always recruiting the same muscle fibers, in the same ways, resulting in limited gains of muscle, strength, and definition. You can take the same exercise and just by altering it a bit, you'll involve different muscle fibers, thereby increasing stimulation and results! Take a classic lower body exercise—the squat. You can perform a narrow or wide legged squat; perform the squat on the floor, on an unstable surface such as the BOSU; or perform a One-Legged Squat to add balance. These will all challenge and recruit different muscle fibers. Other ways to add variety with the same exercise is to alternate using machines and free weights. In your Buns and Legs Workout, you'll find a number of variations of classic lower body exercises such as the squat and lunge.

ALL ABOUT BALANCE

One really important concept we want to stress is the importance of equally training opposing muscle groups (agonists and antagonists). The hamstrings and quadriceps are opposing muscles, as are the inner and outer thighs (the adductors and abductors). It is important that you not overtrain one muscle group while neglecting its opposite, because doing so leaves you vulnerable to injury (and you'll look odd too!). You'll find that the workouts in this book ensure that you pay attention to balancing your workout so that your entire lower body is firm and strong.

Often women clients come to us fearing that if they work out with weights their legs will get too big, that they'll end up with "thunder thighs." We assure you that it is exceedingly difficult and virtually impossible for average women to build up their legs to that point. A sensible weight training regimen for the legs, which involves working the muscles to fatigue, will not give you huge legs, but will give you beautifully defined, sculpted, shapely legs. We don't know many women who don't want that! There also is no way to actually spot reduce the fat from your thighs. You can do leg lifts all day long for a year and the only way you'll lose the extra fat on your legs is to perform cardiovascular exercise. The cardiovascular exercise will burn the fat throughout your physique. Weight training will define the muscles underneath the fat and alter the shape of your lower body. Once you have added muscle to your lower body you also will experience a rise in your metabolic rate because muscle requires more energy than fat at rest. Once you reach the section containing our recommended routines, you'll notice that we suggest doing sufficient cardiovascular exercise each week. When your fitness goals include losing excess fat on your lower body, we recommend that you perform cardiovascular exercise for 20 to 40 minutes three to six times a week, in addition to sculpting your lower body with the Buns and Legs Workout.

Another note on balance: while many women are primarily concerned with their abdominals and lower body, it is important that exercises for the upper body, along with cardiovascular exercise, be included in your overall fitness program to ensure a well-balanced, strong, and fit overall body. Too many women neglect to train their upper bodies adequately (they may do a push-up here and there, or some light shoulder training). This potentially results in having beautifully defined legs, but a flabby or skinny upper body—something that becomes readily apparent in the hot days of summer when you are wearing shoulder-baring tops or swimwear. A beautiful body is a well-balanced and toned body from head to toe. For this reason, you'll find that in the workout sections we also suggest that you do exercises for your upper body, which can be found in *The Body Sculpting Bible,* on your off days.

This book also features a workout for your abdominals, pelvis and lower back (your body's core). The abdominals include the rectus abdominis, the outer abs, which start at the sternum and rib cage and insert on the pubic bone. These muscles flex your spine. The abs also are comprised of the external and internal obliques, which you use when you twist and lean, and the transverse abdominis, which lies deep within the abdominal wall, and plays a crucial role in stabilization.

EQUIPMENT NEEDED

Because this program focuses on building lean muscle, shape, and definition in your butt and legs, the workout routines primarily utilize dumbbell-based exercises as well as some machine exercises. There's been a lot of debate in recent years as to whether free weights are "better" than machines. The best answer is that machines, free weights, and balance equipment all are great, and which you should use depends upon your goals, on your level of fitness, and on your likes. Here are some of the distinguishing characteristics of each method of training:

Free weight exercises recruit the most muscle fibers, so in order to get faster results, free-weights are preferable. Why? Your body is designed to be in a three-dimensional universe—we move in three planes: the sagittal (flexion and extension), transverse (internal and external rotation), and frontal (abduction and adduction). Free-weight training allows your body to move in a three-dimensional environment and involves not only training for a specific muscle group, but also balance, stability, and core training as well.

Whenever you use a machine, you limit your body to a two-dimensional universe and consequently you limit the number of muscle fibers that are going to do work. However, machines often are safer and easier to use, especially for a newcomer to strength training. They are also fabulous if you have an injury and still want to work out. For example, you may have a strain in your lower back, which would make doing free-weight squats painful and dangerous. Instead, you can perform the leg press, using the Leg Press on Machine, which alleviates additional strain on your lower back. Machines also are great for isolating certain muscle groups that are hard to reach with conventional free weights (such as the curling action of a hamstrings). In the end, as we always stress, variety is the spice of exercise. Mix them up; use machines, free-weights, and other equipment to keep your muscles and your mind constantly challenged in different ways.

We also include several exercises that utilize a fitness ball. These are large inflatable balls that you use to perform core and strengthening exercises. You can purchase a ball at any sports store or online. These balls have grown tremendously in popularity during the last decade. They are great because they incorporate stability, posture, balance, and core training—thereby involving greater recruitment of muscle fibers. Small, firmer balls are more challenging than larger, soft balls. If you are deconditioned you may want to start with a larger, soft ball until you've built up your core strength and stability. In general, the size ball you choose depends on your height: If you are under 5 feet, the American Council on Exercise recommends using a ball that is 45 cm in diameter. If you are taller than 5 feet, select one that is 55 cm in diameter. For some exercises, there is an option to use the BOSU (Both Sides Under) ball, a dome-shaped training device that integrates balance and core stabilization, which is increasingly becoming a common piece of equipment in gyms.

SELECTING WEIGHT

The weight you select for each exercise depends on the number of repetitions that you need to do for a particular set. First some definitions: A **rep, or repetition,** is performing an exercise (for example a hamstring curl) one time. A **set** is made up of a given number of repetitions of the same exercise (for example, a set of lunges may consist of 12 reps). In general, you want to keep your repetition range between 8 and 20 maximum. Research shows that the greatest strength and sculpting gains occur when you perform 8 to 15 repetitions of an exercise with weight that is heavy enough to make you feel that you cannot do another **repetition** at the end of the set. This is called the point of **muscular failure**—weight training

is one of the few activities in life where you succeed when you fail!

So, if you need to do 10 to 12 repetitions for one set, you need to pick a weight where you fail (the point at which completing another repetition in good form becomes impossible) between 10 and 12 reps. This takes a bit of practice, but after a while you will become extremely accurate at choosing the correct weight for a particular repetition range. If you pick a weight that allows you to do more than 12 repetitions, you'll need to increase the amount of weight being lifted on the next set. If you reach failure before hitting the tenth rep, you'll need to decrease the amount of weight being lifted. So when you get to the point where you can no longer lift a particular weight for a pre-determined repetition range, simply decrease the weight and prepare yourself for the next set. Conversely, when you are unable to reach failure within the prescribed repetition range on a set, it is time to increase the weight on the next set, preferably in small increments.

Reaching failure is really important to realizing strength and sculpting gains. Do not be afraid to use weight that's heavy enough to allow you to reach failure. Remember, a woman's body does not produce enough testosterone, the male hormone responsible for creating huge amounts of muscle. You will not get huge. You will build beautifully lean and toned muscle tissue that lifts your butt and lengthens your legs.

In the past, people were told to determine their one-rep-maximum (which is the heaviest weight you can lift once and only once) and then work at 60 to 80 percent of that weight. This is dangerous, however, since you may lift weight that is way too heavy while trying to determine your one-rep maximum. Instead of trying to find your one rep max we advise you to select your weights based on the number of repetitions prescribed by parameters in the workout program.

LIFTING TECHNIQUES

PROPER BREATHING

The correct way to breathe while performing an exercise is to exhale (breathe out) while you are forcing the weight up (the concentric phase, or muscle contraction) and to inhale (breathe in) while you are lowering or releasing the weight (the eccentric phase, or the negative portion of the exercise). For example, if you are doing a leg extension, exhale while you extend your legs and inhale while bending them. When performing a squat, you exhale as you lift up and inhale as you bend your legs and lower your body. If you are lifting heavy weight, be careful that you don't inadvertently hold your breath.

SPEED OF LIFTING

While there has been interest recently in very slow lifting of weights, we have found that it is good only for beginners who are new to weight lifting. It helps them to learn and master the movement and prevents them from using bad exercise form. However, as you become more advanced, science and our own experience indicate that you should lift the weight as quickly as possible without sacrificing form and without involving momentum (jerking and bouncing of the weights). You create more force by lifting faster and therefore more muscle fibers need to be activated. If you do not use momentum to help move the weight, you can be sure that the force you generate during the movement is created solely by your muscles. This is what helps stimulate your muscles to grow, creating the tone and shape that you so desire. While some believe that super-slow lifting is beneficial because it is difficult to perform and painful, it is not the best way to stimulate muscle growth. Super-slow lifting generates too much lactic acid within your muscles and fatigues them before they reach real momentary muscular failure.

Science tells us that Force = Mass (in this case the weight you are lifting) times Acceleration (the speed at which you lift the weight). Therefore, the best way to lift weights is to lift them at a relatively fast rate (approximately four seconds to perform each rep) with total control of the weight and no use of momentum. Since you won't be jerking the weights or using shaky movements during exercise, the risk of getting injured is no greater than the risk of getting injured lifting super slowly.

A couple of last things about lifting speed:

1. The eccentric part of the movement, or the part where the weight is lowered (as when you straighten your leg out of a hamstring curl) needs to be per-

formed in a slower, more controlled manner. Research indicates that the negative portion of the movement is of utmost importance for strength and mass gains. Also, an accelerated movement on the eccentric portion could lead to injury.

2. If you are lifting a weight that allows you to do only 8 repetitions, it will look like you are lifting the weight slowly even though you are lifting it as fast as possible. This is because the heavier weight is more difficult to move, even though you are trying to accelerate as fast as you can.

THE PROGRAM

The Buns & Legs Workout is a six-week program consisting of three workouts each week for the beginner phase, four workouts for the intermediate phase and six workouts for the advanced phase. On the beginner phase, two of the three workouts focus on the musculature of the lower body. In the intermediate phase, two of the four workouts also focus on the lower body, and in the advanced workout, three out of six workouts accentuate the lower body. Consider yourself a beginner if you are new to weight training or have been training for less than three months. Use the intermediate program if you have three months to under one year of weight training. Otherwise, you can try the challenging advanced program. These workouts are performed on non-consecutive days, thus allowing 48 hours of rest between your workouts to facilitate recovery in the muscles. When you work out you create tiny tears in the muscles, and when these tears repair, growth occurs. If you work out the same muscles on consecutive days, you do not allow for muscle repair, and you inhibit gains. Remember, ladies: Results are not achieved while you work out. Your rest days are what actually yield results. However, this only works when you've worked hard enough to activate those rebuilding components. Work hard and rest hard!

The three workouts in the Buns & Legs Workout use the program technique known as periodization, which involves varying your strength-training program in 14-day intervals in order to prevent your body from adapting. In order for your muscles to continue to be challenged and for your body to keep realizing benefits, it needs to be surprised a bit—otherwise, you will find yourself at a plateau point where you are no longer getting leaner, or more sculpted. There are many ways that a program can be varied. For example, you can change the types and order of exercises, the number of repetitions and sets you perform for each exercise, the order in which you perform the exercises, the speed of lifting, and the amount of rest time between exercises. Periodization varies your workout in a logical and orderly manner in order to deliver the fastest results possible. Studies consistently show that people who train using the periodization approach realize greater gains than those whose routines remain the same.

Tied closely to the periodization concept is the principle of progression. In order for you to make any muscular gains, and to change the appearance of a muscle, you need to progress—that is, constantly present your muscles with a challenge. Progression includes many things, such as increasing the weight that you lift, or the number of repetitions, or the rest between sets, or the number of sets that you do in order to increase the overall load on your body. To be effective and safe, you must progress slowly and rationally. Do not suddenly increase your weight load by a great amount. Test it out. See how heavy you can go and still maintain proper form, and perform the desired number of reps where you reach failure by the time you reach the end of a set.

Progression can also lead to an increased use of dumbbells and less reliance on machines as your balance and kinesthetic awareness improve, and as you gain enough strength to perform a free-weight exercise in good form.

You will find that the workouts in this book are different on each day of the week, and that every two weeks, the workout changes in other, bigger ways, including the number of reps/sets you perform and the amount of rest time in between exercises. The way it changes depends on whether you are doing the Beginner, Intermediate, or Advanced version. For some two-week segments you might be performing **modified compound supersets**—back-to-back exercises for opposing muscle groups (for example your hamstrings and quadriceps) with the prescribed rest period in between each set. For the following two-week periods you might switch to **supersetting**—when you perform two exercises back-to-back without any rest in between. Finally, the biggest challenge comes from performing **giant sets**—four exercises performed one after the other with no rest in between each exercise (Note: The only rest time occurs at the end of the fourth set, before you cycle back to the first exercise.) All three Buns & Legs Workouts also include abdominal and cardiovascular components.

HOW TO INCORPORATE THE BUNS & LEGS WORKOUT INTO *THE BODY SCULPTING BIBLE* WORKOUTS

There are several ways you can use the workouts presented in this book. If you are already following the 14-Day Body Sculpting Program from the original *Body Sculpting Bible for Women,* then just substitute the lower body workouts for the workouts presented in Part III of this book, once you finish the 6-week Body Sculpting Cycle of the original workout. Please refer to Part III of this book for more details as to how to incorporate the workouts in your existing Body Sculpting Bible Program.

If this is the first book that you have purchased from the Body Sculpting Bible series, please make sure that you incorporate upper body workouts on the days advised in Part III of this book so that you do not create an imbalanced physique.

ZONE-TONE FOR MAXIMUM RESULTS

We are strong advocates of using a technique that we've developed—called the Zone-Tone method—to maximize your fitness gains. This method uses the mind-to-muscle connection, coupled with proper exercise technique and form, in order to most effectively stimulate your muscle fibers during an exercise. It involves really thinking about the muscles you are training right before you perform an exercise. In so doing, you increase mental focus and pre-isolate specific muscles.

To Zone-Tone:

1. **Zone in on the individual muscles you are training before each exercise.** Concentrate on the muscle, mentally tensing and contracting (flexing) it as hard as you can before you actually begin the contraction. Here is where you engage and begin making the mind-to-muscle connection.

2. **Maintain your mind-to-muscle connection during the execution of the exercise:** Throughout the execution of the exercise, deliberately feel the muscle elongate (stretch) and contract (or flex), as you move along from point A to point B (The full range of movement for a particular exercise). In other words, contract (flex) the muscle as hard as you can in the same way that you did in step one, but with the exception that now you'll have a weight in your hand, plus add movement. When you effectively communicate with a specific muscle and

prepare it for the upcoming set (work load), you have successfully engaged the mind-to-muscle connection. By keeping this connection active throughout the duration of the exercise, just that one set can produce the results of five sets! Do you realize what this can do for you? If you implement these principles in your training regimen, you can undoubtedly create unbelievably toned and incredibly defined muscles in half the time!

HOW TO FURTHER ENHANCE ZONE-TONE'S EFFECT

Here is a way to compound your Zone-Tone effect with little or no additional time expenditure.

When you're getting ready for bed at night, before you get too sleepy, take this very opportune time to practice the following protocol: as you begin to relax, start with your feet and focus on your toes. Slightly wiggle them and concentrate on feeling even the slightest movement in each individual toe. As you move on from the feet toward your knees and up, zone in on every body part along the way. Now here's where it can get tricky. Simply focusing on the individual muscles of the body is not enough, because you cannot truly get a feel for how they feel when they are in motion.

To help you home in and actually gain a feel for each of these muscles, do the following:

- As you get to each individual body part, stop and contract the muscle as

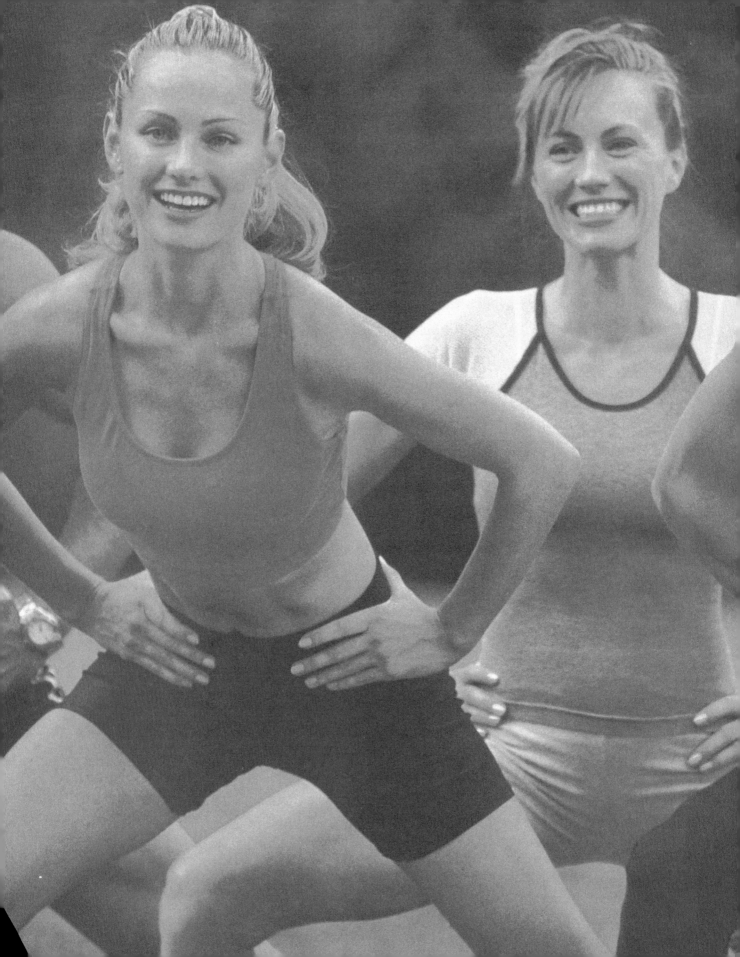

well as you can. Do this three to five times and then relax. Hold each contraction for about 3 to 5 seconds and then relax for 5 seconds before you begin the next cycle.

- Remember the exact area where you felt the intended muscle contract and now focus all of your attention and energy on relaxing that very same area. This teaches you to be in complete control of your entire superficial muscular system and will give you the opportunity to realize maximum muscular efficiency.

Here is yet another technique you should use to further enhance the overall effects of the Zone-Tone method:

After you complete each set of an exercise, stand in the mirror and contract (flex) the muscles that you were exercising as hard as you can and hold for a count of 3 to 5 seconds. This will help you to create a stronger mind-to-muscle connection and accurately identify and call upon those individual muscles during exercise. In addition, it will help to bring more blood and nutrients to the intended muscle, for enhanced results.

We can't tell you enough how important it is to practice the Zone-Tone method both when you're working out and also while at rest. As with anything, the more you practice the Zone-Tone method the quicker and more powerful it will become. Soon you will realize, first hand, the astonishing results gained from this powerful concept. Good luck, train hard, and get in the zone!

WORKING OUT AND YOUR PERIOD

There's no reason to let your monthly periods disrupt your workout schedule. Most women find that they can maintain their regular activity levels throughout their periods. If you usually suffer from PMS, and cramps in particular, you'll probably find that exercising actually helps to alleviate your symptoms, because it releases tension in your body. A particularly good exercise to perform if you suffer from cramps is a pelvic tilt, where you lie on your back—with your knees bent and your feet on the floor—and lift your buttocks up, then rock gently back and forth. If you tend to feel faint at times, especially when your period is heavy, you may want to avoid exercises in an inverted position (when your head is lower than your chest). On those days when your symptoms are severe, don't forgo your workout, but take it down a notch in intensity (for example, if you run for cardiovascular exercise, you may opt to walk fast instead). As always, make sure you have plenty of water to drink before, during, and after your session.

Also bear in mind that exercise, through its release of natural opiates, helps to elevate your mood and can alleviate PMS-related "blues" or feelings of depression that many women experience.

One word of caution: Overly strenuous exercising is never recommended. It can lead to hormonal alterations that can disrupt your menstrual cycle and even cause its cessation (amenorrhea). If you find that you are becoming obsessive about your workouts, are working out for more than 90 minutes each session, and have body fat levels below 10 percent, you are at risk for amenorrhea.

KNOW YOUR GOALS

Without goals you are like a ship on the middle of the sea, just drifting away with no sense of direction. In order to achieve success we need to clearly define and ingrain our goals in our minds. Otherwise, like the drifting boat, if you get anywhere it will be by mere chance. Here are some tips for successful goal setting.

- **WRITE DOWN YOUR GOALS:** If they are in writing they will be clear and you can always return to them when you need reinforcement.

- **BE SPECIFIC:** what measurements do you want to have? What about your body-fat percentage and total body weight? How sculpted do you want your muscles to be?

- **MAKE GOALS REALISTIC AND ATTAINABLE WITHIN THE TIMEFRAME:** If you have a large-frame body type, going from a size 12 to a size 4 in six weeks may be unreasonable. Know your body. Set yourself up for success, not failure.

For the next six weeks I will:

Lose	_____	pounds of fat
Gain	_____	pounds of muscle
Weigh	_____	pounds

Have measurements of:

| Hips | _____ | inches |
| Thighs | _____ | inches |

WORKING OUT DURING PREGNANCY AND MENOPAUSE

Pregnancy and menopause, two major life stages of great hormonal changes for women, present some workout considerations. Here are some guidelines for working out while pregnant:

- Consult with your ob/gyn about the exercise program you are about to undertake.

- Work out at a moderate intensity (you should not get too over-heated or ever exercise to the point of exhaustion).

- Extended warmups and cooldowns are essential.

- Listen to your body—if it doesn't feel good, don't do it.

- During the second and third trimesters, avoid exercises in the supine position, as this can cut off nutrients from the fetus.

- Avoid exercise that involves deep flexion or extension (such as going into a deep squat) or quick changes in direction, because your joints are more unstable during pregnancy.

During perimenopause (the months or years leading up to menopause) and menopause (when you have stopped having your period for a full year), your body changes in major ways—particularly with regard to your body's levels of estrogen. Decreased levels of estrogen can lead to feelings of fatigue, mood changes, hot flashes, night sweats, insomnia, and weight gain—especially around

One note: If you are pregnant and beyond your first trimester, it is recommended that you modify all exercises, including those for abdominals, so that you do not perform them in a supine position (lying on your back). When using the ball, select a position with your head and chest lifted, which enables you to perform the exercise without lying fully back on the ball. In addition, as your pregnancy progresses, ball exercises may become too difficult and risky because of changes in your body's equilibrium and balance.

the abdominal area. Exercise can help you to alleviate many of these symptoms as well as protect you from heart disease and osteoporosis (all diseases for which menopausal women are at greater risk). Here are some tips for training:

• Weight training at least twice a week is imperative to help prevent bone loss, fight the flabby effects of gravity, maintain good posture, and prevent injury by increasing strength, balance, and kinesthetic awareness.

• Incorporate more cardiovascular training to offset the weight-gain from a slowing metabolism and to produce endorphins (natural mood-elevating opiates), which are released during aerobic exercise.

• Eat healthfully; consume a diet that consists of plenty of antioxidant-rich vegetables and fruits, is low in fat, high in fiber, and which contains at least 400 mg of calcium a day.

• On days when you are feeling especially tired, take it a bit easier on yourself. Work out hard on the days you feel strong.

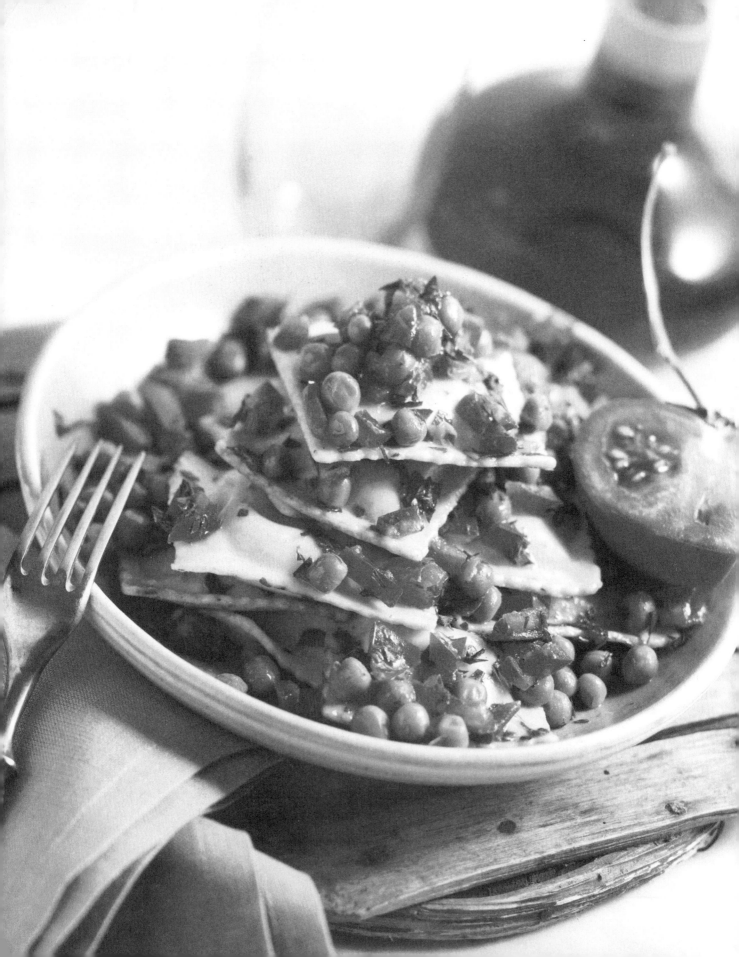

Chapter 2
Optimal Eating

In order to make impressive changes in your lower body, nutrition and training need to go hand in hand. It is a myth that you can eat as much as you want as long as you exercise. We wish that statement were true as much as you do. However, even the most rigorous exercise regimen will be undone by poor eating habits.

The nutritional approach that we find most effective for most healthy women is based on a principle of balance among the major nutrients that your body requires. However, some people, like diabetics, may have unique needs, so it is wise to check with a nutritionist or your doctor before radically changing your eating habits.

That said, the following guidelines and information will help you to formulate a diet that is rich in energy-producing nutrients, and that will support and enhance all

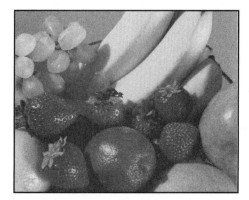

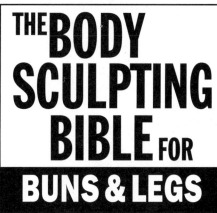

THE **BODY SCULPTING BIBLE** FOR
BUNS & LEGS

2

the hard work you're doing on the Buns & Legs Workout.

NECESSARY NUTRIENTS

There are three macronutrients that the human body needs in order to function properly: carbohydrates, proteins, and fats.

CARBOHYDRATES

Carbohydrates are your body's main source of energy. When you ingest carbohydrates your pancreas releases a hormone called insulin. Insulin is very important because:

- It grabs the carbohydrates and either stores them in the muscle or stores them as fat.
- It grabs the amino acids (protein) and shelters them inside the muscle cells

where they are used for recovery and repair.

Most overweight people on low-fat/high-carbohydrate diets eat an overabundance of carbohydrates. Too many carbohydrates cause a huge release of insulin. When there is too much insulin in the body, your body turns into a fat-storing machine. Therefore, it is important that we eat the right amount and kinds of carbohydrates.

Carbohydrates are divided into complex carbohydrates and simple carbohydrates. The complex carbohydrates provide sustained energy ("timed release") while the simple carbohydrates gives you immediate energy. It is recommended that you eat mainly complex carbohydrates throughout the day, except after your workout when your body needs simple carbohydrates in order to replenish its

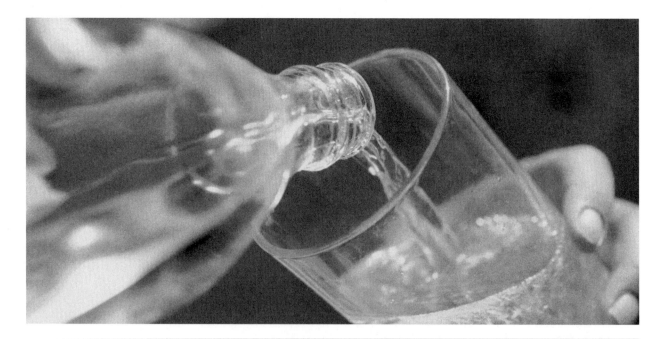

glycogen levels immediately, in order to help muscles recover and rebuild quickly.

There are two types of **complex carbohydrates:** starchy, such as those found in oatmeal, sweet potatoes, and grits; and fibrous, which are plentiful in broccoli, cauliflower, and zucchini. Examples of simple carbohydrates that are healthy include many fruits: apples, bananas, grapes, and oranges.

PROTEIN

Every tissue in your body (i.e., muscle, hair, skin, and nails) is made from protein. Proteins are the building blocks of muscle tissue. Every time you eat protein your metabolism increases by approximately 20 percent. In addition, protein enables carbohydrates to be time released, providing you with sustained energy throughout the day.

In a weight-training program such as the Buns & Legs Workout, you should consume between 1 to 1.5 grams of protein per pound of lean body mass (meaning that if you are 100 lbs, and have 10% body fat, you should consume approximately 90 g of protein since your lean body mass = 90 lb.). Consuming more than 1.5 grams of protein per pound of lean body mass is not recommended.

Good examples of protein are eggs, chicken breast (cooked, skinless and boneless: 6 oz), turkey (cooked, skinless and boneless: 6 oz), lean (90% lean) red meats (6 oz), and tuna (6 oz). Each serving size equals approximately 35 to 40 grams of protein.

FATS

There are three types of fats: saturated, polyunsaturated, and monounsaturated.

Saturated fats are associated with heart disease and high cholesterol levels. They are found to a large extent in products of animal origin. However, some vegetable fats are altered in a way that increases the amount of saturated fats in them by a chemical process known as hydrogenation. Hydrogenated vegetable oils are generally found in packaged foods, and these oils should be avoided at all costs as they have been shown to play a huge role in causing insulin resistance, clogged arteries, and obesity. In addition, coconut oil, palm oil, and palm kernel oil, which are also frequently used in packaged foods, and non-dairy creamers are also highly saturated.

Polyunsaturated fats do not have an effect in cholesterol levels. Most of the fats in vegetable oils, such as canola, corn, cottonseed, safflower, soybean, and sunflower oils, are polyunsaturated. Flaxseed oil, and fish oils are also polyunsaturated. These last two should be the main source of your polyunsaturated fat consumption. If you use flaxseed oil, make sure that it is bottled in a dark container that protects it from light. Also make sure to keep it refrigerated, as heat makes it rancid (therefore never cook with it). These last two fats are usually high in the essential fatty acids and may have antioxidant properties. Corn oil, on the other hand should, never be used for cooking as it contributes to increases in the size of fat cells.

Monounsaturated fats have a health-enhancing effect because they lower the levels of LDL (bad cholesterol) and increase the levels of HDL (good cholesterol). Sources of these fats are extra virgin olive oil and nuts such as cashews, pecans and almonds. Peanut butter fits in here too, but it is really a bean rather than a nut. The main source of your monounsaturated fats should be canned extra virgin olive oil.

We recommend that 20 percent of your calories come from good fats. Any less than 20% and your hormonal production decreases. Any more than 20% and you start accumulating plenty of fat. Good sources of fat are extra virgin olive oil from a can (1 tablespoon), natural peanut butter (2 tablespoons), flaxseed oil (1 tablespoon), and fish oils (1 tablespoon). Each serving size contains approximately 14 grams of fat.

In our approach to nutrition, we use a diet that contains all of the macronutrients in a more balanced manner. The breakdown of the nutrient looks like this:

40% Carbs

40% Protein

20% Fats

NOTE: If you are pregnant, bear in mind that during your second and third trimesters you require an additional 300 calories per day without exercise.† Therefore, if you are exercising during your pregnancy, make sure you consume enough calories to get the nutrition you and your baby need. Consult your physician or a nutritionist.

CHARACTERISTICS OF A GOOD NUTRITION PROGRAM

- **YOUR NUTRITION PLAN SHOULD BE BASED ON EATING SMALL AND FREQUENT MEALS THROUGHOUT THE DAY.** Aim for eating five or six small meals each day, rather than a couple of large ones.

- **ALL MEALS SHOULD CONTAIN CARBOHYDRATES, PROTEIN AND FAT IN THE CORRECT RATIOS.** Balancing each meal ensures that your body is fueled with energy in the proper proportion to maximize power.

- **DO NOT SMOKE AND LIMIT ALCOHOL CONSUMPTION.** Smoking is just plain horrible for you, and alcohol can lead to increased fat gain as each gram of alcohol has 7 calories. To make matters worse, alcohol not only increases your blood sugar levels, which in turn signals the body to produce insulin (too much insulin protects fat from being burned), but once your blood sugar goes down again your appetite will go up. Not good when you are trying to get in shape.

- **HYDRATE FREQUENTLY.** Nearly 65 percent of our bodies are composed of water. It is always important to make sure you drink enough, especially if you are working out. A good rule of thumb is to multiply your body-weight times .66 in ounces of water per day. So for instance, if you weigh 120 lbs, then you need to consume around 79 ounces of water per day.

IMPORTANCE OF CALCIUM

As a woman, it is essential that you get adequate amounts of calcium—from 400 to 800 mg per day. The mineral, which is found in dark green vegetables like broccoli and spinach, as well as in dairy products such as yogurt and milk, helps to increase bone mass, and can help prevent osteoporosis, the bone-thinning disease common in mid-life women. Although osteoporosis may not manifest until a woman has gone through menopause, research indicates that prevention should begin when a woman is in her twenties and thirties. In addition, diets rich in calcium—especially calcium from dairy—have been linked to healthier body weights. Women on the same calorie diets with different amounts of calcium were studied and those who had more calcium from dairy products lost more weight. Experts theorize that calcium may suppress levels of the substance 1.25-dihydroxyvitamin D, which stimulates fat production in the body.

CALORIC NEEDS

Caloric requirements for most women fluctuate between 1,200 and 1,500 calories per day. However, if you eat the same number of calories day in and day out, your body will adapt to that amount and you will stop losing fat. To prevent this, we recommend that you alternate between 1,200 and 1,500 calories; for two weeks consume 1,200 calories and then the following two weeks you consume 1,500. Note: If you are pregnant, or trying to become preg-

---

1,200-CALORIE WEEK MACRONUTRIENT REQUIREMENTS

120 grams of carbohydrates (mostly complex, with simple carbs being saved for after the workout)
120 grams of protein
26 grams of fats

In five meals that comes out to approximately:
24 grams of carbs per meal
24 grams of protein per meal
5 grams of fats per meal

1,500-CALORIE WEEK MACRONUTRIENT REQUIREMENTS

150 grams of carbohydrates (mostly complex, with simple carbs being saved for after the workout)
150 grams of protein
33 grams of fats

In six meals that comes out to approximately:
25 grams of carbs per meal
25 grams of protein per meal
6 grams of fats per meal

---

nant, it is imperative that you consult your doctor about your nutritional needs and the exercise program that makes the most sense for you.

Once you know the total number of calories you need to take in every day, calculate the amount (in grams) of each nutrient by using the percentages above in the following formula:

Total amount of carbs for the day = (total number of calories x 0.40)/4

Total amount of protein for the day = (total number of calories x 0.40)/4

Total amount of fat for the day = (total number of calories x 0.20)/9

NOTE: Carbs and protein are divided by 4 because there are 4 calories per gram of carbs or of protein. For fats, we divide by 9 since there are 9 calories for every gram of fat).

Divide all of the results from the formulas above by 5 (By 6 if you are eating 6 times a day) to obtain the amount of each nutrient that you will need to consume at each meal.

The next section features a chart indicating what specific foods to eat at each meal.

CHOOSING FOOD

One of the biggest challenges that we face when starting a diet is deciding what to eat every day. Now that you have calculated the amount of carbs, protein, and fats you need for each meal, you need to choose which foods to eat. For this purpose the food-groups table found on the next page contains the food values for the foods we recommend you eat. It is very accurate. However, if you happen to discover a discrepancy between the nutritional information on a food label and the chart, use the information from the food label.

The following chart indicates the types and quantities of foods to choose for each one of your meals. The times are, of course, approximate and you can change them based on your own schedule. The post-workout meal assumes that you are training in the morning, but if this is not the case, have some complex carbs in the morning and move the post workout meal to after your workout.

1,200-CALORIE WEEKS

MEAL 1 (7:30 AM)-BREAKFAST (POST-WORKOUT)
CHOOSE 24 GRAMS FROM GROUP A
CHOOSE 24 GRAMS FROM GROUP C

MEAL 2 (10:30 AM)-MORNING BREAK SNACK
CHOOSE 24 GRAMS FROM GROUP A
CHOOSE 24 GRAMS FROM GROUP B

MEAL 3 (1:30 PM)-LUNCH TIME
CHOOSE 24 GRAMS FROM GROUP A
CHOOSE 19 GRAMS FROM GROUP B
CHOOSE 5 GRAMS FROM GROUP D

MEAL 4 (3:30 PM)-AFTERNOON BREAK SNACK
CHOOSE 24 GRAMS FROM GROUP A
CHOOSE 24 GRAMS FROM GROUP B

MEAL 5 (6:30 PM)-DINNER
CHOOSE 24 GRAMS FROM GROUP A
CHOOSE 14 GRAMS FROM GROUP B
CHOOSE 10 GRAMS FROM GROUP D

1,500-CALORIE WEEKS

MEAL 1 (7:30 AM)-BREAKFAST (POST-WORKOUT)
CHOOSE 25 GRAMS FROM GROUP A
CHOOSE 25 GRAMS FROM GROUP C

MEAL 2 (10:30 AM)-MORNING BREAK SNACK
CHOOSE 25 GRAMS FROM GROUP A
CHOOSE 25 GRAMS FROM GROUP B

MEAL 3 (12:30 PM)-LUNCH TIME
CHOOSE 25 GRAMS FROM GROUP A
CHOOSE 20 GRAMS FROM GROUP B
CHOOSE 5 GRAMS FROM GROUP D

MEAL 4 (3:30 PM)-AFTERNOON BREAK SNACK
CHOOSE 25 GRAMS FROM GROUP A
CHOOSE 25 GRAMS FROM GROUP B

MEAL 5 (6:30 PM)-DINNER
CHOOSE 25 GRAMS FROM GROUP A
CHOOSE 15 GRAMS FROM GROUP B
CHOOSE 10 GRAMS FROM GROUP D

MEAL 6 (8:30 PM)-LATE SNACK
CHOOSE 25 GRAMS FROM GROUP A
CHOOSE 15 GRAMS FROM GROUP B
CHOOSE 10 GRAMS FROM GROUP D

NOTE: Include one tsp of olive oil three times a day with any meals (except the post-workout meal) on one day. The next day, include one tsp of olive oil once a day and one tsp of flaxseed oil twice a day with any meals (except the post-workout meal). This, in conjunction with the naturally occurring fats in the food, will cover your essential fats needs.

NOTE: Include one tsp of olive oil three times a day with any meals (except the post-workout meal) on one day. The next day, include one tsp of olive oil once a day and one tsp of flax oil twice a day with any meals (except the post-workout meal). This, in conjunction with the naturally occurring fats in the food will cover your essential fats needs.

FOOD GROUP TABLES

For the post-workout meal (meal that comes after the workout is performed), choose one item from Group A and one item from Group C in order to create a balanced meal. For all other meals, choose one item from Group A, one item from Group B, and one item from Group D in order to create a balanced meal. Remember to adjust the serving size depending upon the amount of nutrients that you require per meal.

GROUP A : PROTEINS

FOOD	GRAMS	FOOD	GRAMS
Chicken breast (3.5 oz. broiled)	35	Whitefish (3.5 oz broiled)	31
Tuna fish (spring water) 3.5 oz	35	Halibut (3.5 oz broiled)	31
Turkey breast (3.5 oz broiled)	28	Cod (3.5 oz broiled)	31
Whey protein (2 scoops)	20	Round steak (3.5 oz broiled)	33

GROUP B : COMPLEX CARBOHYDRATE

FOOD	GRAMS	FOOD	GRAMS
Baked potato (3.5 oz)	21	Rice (white or brown) 2/3 cup	31
Plain oatmeal (1/2 cup dry)	27	Shredded wheat (1 cup dry)	31
Plain pasta (1 cup)	44	Corn (1/2 cup)	31
Whole-wheat bread (1 slice)	12	Yams (3 oz roasted or baked)	21

GROUP C : SIMPLE CARBOHYDRATE

FOOD	GRAMS	FOOD	GRAMS
Apple (1 fruit)	15	Banana (6 oz)	27
Cantaloupe (1 fruit)	25	Grapes (1 cup)	14
Strawberries (1 cup)	9	Yogurt (1 serving)	27

GROUP D : FIBROUS CARBOHYDRATE

FOOD (10 OZ SERVING)	GRAMS	FOOD (10 OZ SERVING)	GRAMS
Asparagus	25	Squash	25
Broccoli	25	Green Beans	25
Cabbage	25	Cauliflower	25
Celery	25	Cucumber	25
Mushrooms	25	Lettuce	25
Red or Green Peppers	25	Tomato	25
Spinach	25	Zucchini	25

SHOULD YOU SUPPLEMENT?

While it is best to obtain all of your nutrients from healthful, fresh foods, you may want to use supplements when you find you're not eating as well as you should. Here are some of our recommendations.

1. A good **multiple vitamin and mineral formula** taken preferably with your post-workout meal or at breakfast on non-workout days in order to avoid any nutritional deficiencies. Make sure that it has at least 500 mg of calcium. Otherwise, get a separate calcium supplement such as calcium citrate, which is best absorbed by the body. Calcium needs vitamin D in order to be absorbed properly.

2. **Chromium picolinate** (200 mcg) also with the post-workout meal or at breakfast. This mineral is good for increasing the cells' acceptance of the hormone insulin. A good insulin sensitivity is necessary in order to have the fat burning process optimized. **Note:** Some multiple vitamin/mineral formulas already have this in them so check the label.

3. 1000 mg of **vitamin C** three times a day. Start with only 500 mg and increase the dosage by 500 mg per week until you reach the 3000 mg total. This is in order to avoid any stomach problems. Vitamin C is fantastic at reducing levels of cortisol, which is the stress hormone released by the adrenal glands that likes to eat muscle and store fat.

4. **Whey protein shakes or meal replacement shakes** like Prolab's Naturally Lean Complex, or any other similar formula, are useful while you are on the go and cannot have a real meal. We recommend ProLab's Lean Mass Complex because it is based on complex carbohydrates and a blend of different proteins consisting of a 40/40/20 macronutrient ratio. It contains 20 grams of carbs, 20 grams of proteins and 4 grams of good fats, making it the perfect meal replacement supplement for this program. The product is also easy to prepare. It requires no blender—just some water and a spoon, and the taste is fantastic.

Part 2

The Exercises

It's time to introduce the exercises that comprise your Buns & Legs Workout. We begin with a chapter on stretching to improve flexibility, and continue with exercises to sculpt your butt and legs. Carefully read the descriptions of each exercise, making recommended modifications to fit your fitness level and goals.

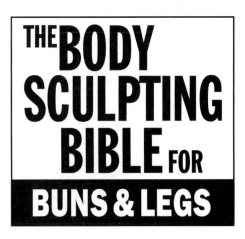

THE BODY SCULPTING BIBLE FOR **BUNS & LEGS**

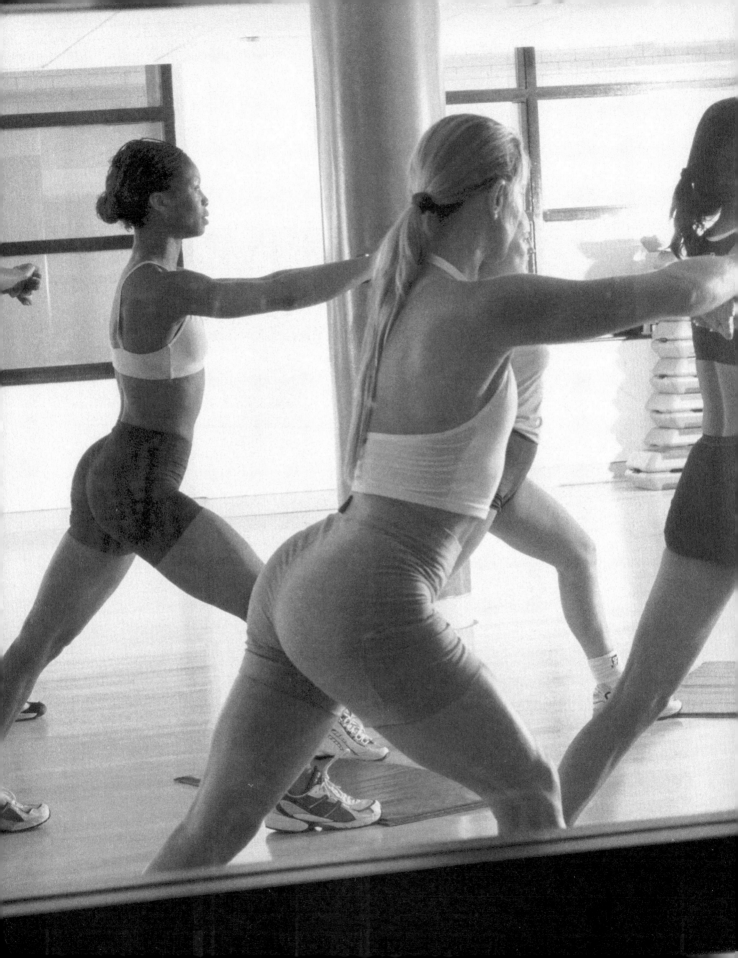

Chapter 3

Sleek Stretching

Many of our clients don't like to take the time to stretch out their muscles. We understand. If you are pressed for time, it is easy to forgo the stretch component of your workout because you feel that it's not doing much of anything. But in fact, the pre-workout warm up and post-workout stretch are vital components of your Buns & Legs Workout. And they don't require a lot of time—just a few minutes. The next few pages will show you how to warm up most effectively for your workout and how to stretch out your muscles to prevent injury.

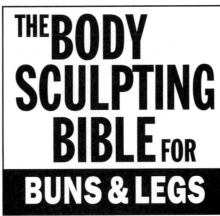

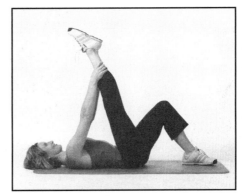

THE BODY SCULPTING BIBLE FOR BUNS & LEGS

ACTIVELY WARM UP BEFORE YOU BEGIN

Research indicates that you should perform an active warm up before you begin a workout. The key word here is active. In the past, people were told to perform holding stretches (called static stretches) before they worked out—for example, stretching your legs before going for a run. However, the most recent research, including one major review of the research on stretching conducted by researchers at SMBD-Jewish General Hospital in Montreal, has found that stretching before you exercise does not prevent injury. (In certain cases, if you stretch right before an activity, you actually increase your risk for injury because the stretch can temporarily reduce force and power in your muscle). Instead, it is recommended that you stretch after your workout to improve your range of motion on a regular basis, a few times a week.

Before you work out you want to increase your heart rate and prepare your body for the work ahead. This is best achieved through an active warmup, which increases blood flow to your muscles preparing your neuromuscular system for the movements you will need to perform.

The best active warm-up for the Buns & Legs Workout consists of about five minutes of movement involving large muscles. For example, a combination of squats (body weight only), jumping jacks, jogging or fast walking, or five minutes on a elliptical trainer. In your warmup you want to try to use all of the lower body muscles you will be working during workout.

It is also very helpful to warmup by emulating some of the actual weight-lifting exercises you will perform during your workout. For example, if your workout is to consist of squats, your warm up could include performing those exercises with little or no weight. This is an effective way to prepare your body and mind for the workout by increasing your kinesthetic awareness and by moving blood to the muscles that will be working. It also enhances safety by providing an opportunity to practice proper form before you perform the exercise with resistance.

While there's scant evidence that static stretching (the type of stretch that involves holding a stretched position for a number of seconds with no bouncing) before your workout prevents injury, you can do a few pre-workout stretches that are dynamic. Dynamic stretches involve performing several repetitions of bringing a muscle quickly into a stretched position and then immediately releasing it. This type of stretching helps to prepare your muscles for the workout ahead.

STATIC STRETCH AT THE END, NOT BEGINNING, OF YOUR WORKOUT

The optimal, safest time to do static stretching is at the end of the workout. This is when your muscles are warm due to increased blood flow that occurred during your workout. Therefore, it is the best time to elongate them. In addition, there's less risk of causing injury by over-stretching when the muscles are warm. In contrast, if you perform static stretches on cold muscles (for example, first thing in the morning, when your muscles are very tight), your range of motion is much more limited and you risk pushing the stretch too far and injuring the muscle or connective tissues. There are two ways you can perform the static stretches in the Buns & Legs Workout. You may opt to perform a stretch for a particular muscle group during your rest period right after you have completed all the sets of exercises for that group (for example, your hamstrings) and before you move on to the next set of exercises. Or you may perform all of the static stretches at the very end of your workout.

THE PROPER WAY TO STRETCH

The way you stretch makes all the difference between an effective, fitness-enhancing stretch and a dangerous one. First, begin your static stretch by inhaling from your diaphragm (the base of your lungs) rather than from your chest (a helpful mental image is to imagine you are inflating a balloon with your breathing). As you move into the stretch position, exhale. Go deep enough into a stretch to feel tension in the muscles you are stretching. Never force a stretch. Hold the stretch position for 10 to 30 seconds before releasing. Continue to breathe deeply while in the stretch position. Never hold your breath. As you hold the stretch, you will begin to feel your muscles moving from a state

of tension to relaxation. At this point, you can try to take the stretch a bit deeper. It is normal to feel some discomfort during the initial moments of the stress; if you feel any pain, however, ease up on the stretch immediately. Ease up on the stretch also if your muscles start to shake; this indicates you are in an overstretched position for your body. During a static stretch you want to hold the stretch without any bouncing (ballistic stretching). While ballistic stretching has its place in preparing the body for some athletic moves, it is not recommended at the end of your Buns & Legs program.

LOWER BODY STRETCH PROGRAM

The stretches that appear on the following pages can be done dynamically before your workout, or statically afterwards. Before your workout, perform several repetitions of each stretch, holding each one for only 1 to 3 seconds. (Also, remember you can simulate the actual exercises you will do in your workout for your warmup.) After your workout, perform one repetition of each stretch but hold without bouncing for as long as 30 seconds.

LYING HAMSTRING STRETCH

This is a great stretch for the backs of your legs, but make sure you don't pull too hard on your leg or take the stretch too far.

TECHNIQUE AND FORM

1 Lie on your back on a mat with your right leg out in front and your left leg bent.

2 Bring your right knee in to your chest, then extend the right leg as straight as possible.

3 Exhale and pull the leg in toward your chest as far as you can, without feeling pain.

4 Lift your upper body to meet the extended leg.

5 Hold for 20 to 30 seconds. As you hold you may find you can increase the range of the stretch.

6 Switch legs.

TRAINER'S TIPS

Try to get the leg you are stretching to form a 90-degree angle with the floor. However, if your leg starts to shake or you feel pain, ease up immediately.

Keeping the opposite leg bent for this stretch relieves pressure on the lower back.

LYING HAMSTRING STRETCH

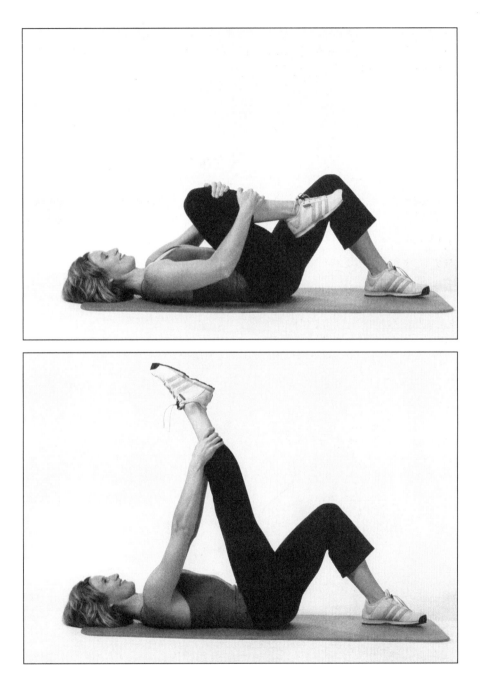

LYING CALF STRETCH

Performing this stretch after the hamstring stretch provides a nice flow.

TECHNIQUE AND FORM

1 Lie on your back with the left leg bent and the right leg straight up in the air.

2 Lift the right leg and then bend it so that your knee comes in to your chest.

3 Gently but firmly hold on to the back of your right thigh with your right hand. With the left hand on the ball of your right foot, press your toes in toward your shin.

4 Hold for 20 to 30 seconds.

5 Switch sides.

TRAINER'S TIPS

Really concentrate on pressing the toes in. To maximize the stretch you may use a towel (drape it around the ball of your foot and pull it in toward you as you stretch.)

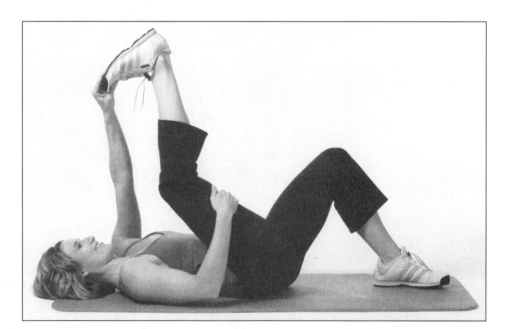

LYING GLUTEAL STRETCH

This stretch relieves tension in the muscles surrounding your butt.

TECHNIQUE AND FORM

1 Lie on your back on a mat with your left leg bent and your right leg extended.

2 Bend the right leg, placing your right ankle against your left thigh.

3 Exhale and lift your left leg off the floor as you pull your hip in toward your chest.

4 Hold for 20 to 30 seconds.

5 Switch sides.

TRAINER'S TIPS

✖ You may try to lift your upper body from the mat as you perform the stretch.

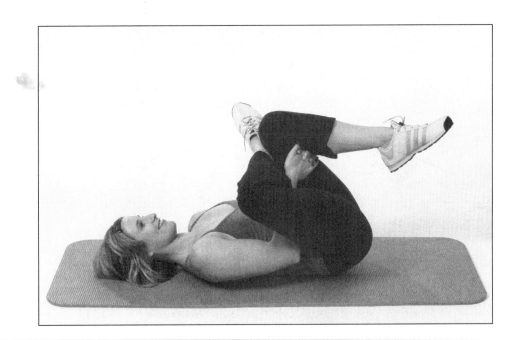

LYING HIP AND THIGH STRETCH

This stretch will release tension in your hip and thighs.

TECHNIQUE AND FORM

1 Lie on your back on a mat with your legs stretched out in front of you and your arms out to the sides.

2 Exhale as you bend one leg over the other, so that the knee of the bent leg comes close to the floor.

3 Use a hand to apply pressure to the bent leg, and to bring the knee closer to the floor.

4 Hold for 20 to 30 seconds.

5 Switch sides.

TRAINER'S TIPS

✪ As you cross the bent leg over the midline of your body, try to keep both shoulders against the floor.

✪ Relax your upper body and breathe deeply into this stretch.

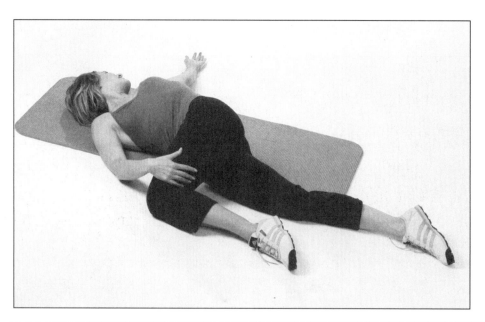

LYING QUADRICEPS STRETCH

When performing this stretch for the fronts of your thighs, make sure you keep your body centered—try not to lean forward or back.

TECHNIQUE AND FORM

1 Lie on your right side with both legs straight out. Bend your left leg back at about a 90-degree angle.

2 Hold on to your left foot with your left hand.

3 Exhale and slowly pull your left leg behind you until you feel a stretch in the front of your thigh.

4 Hold for 20 to 30 seconds.

5 Switch sides.

TRAINER'S TIPS

 Pull your heel in toward your buttocks as much as you can to maximize this stretch.

 You may keep your head down or lifted depending upon what is most comfortable for you and enables you to maintain good form.

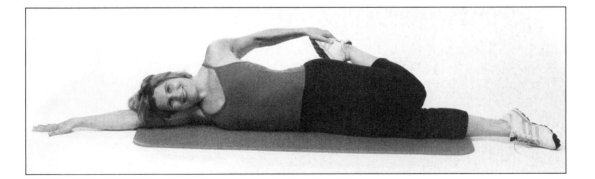

SEATED HAMSTRING STRETCH

Here's another good stretch for the usually tight hamstrings. This stretch also relieves tension in your lower back.

TECHNIQUE AND FORM

1 Sit straight, with your right leg extended in front of you, foot flexed, and your left leg bent so that the heel of your left foot is against your right inner thigh.

2 Interlace your fingers and lift your arms overhead as your inhale.

3 Exhale and slowly bring your arms and torso forward—toward your toes—making sure you initiate the movement from the base of your spine.

4 Go as far forward as you can without feeling pain.

5 Hold for 20 to 30 seconds.

6 Switch sides.

TRAINER'S TIPS

✪ Engage your abdominals as you move into this stretch. This will help you maintain a flat back and improve your range of motion.

✪ Do not push yourself to reach your toes, or to lower your torso too far. Go only as far as you need to feel tension in the back of your legs.

✪ As you hold the stretch for a few seconds, you may find you are able to increase the stretch by lowering your torso a bit more.

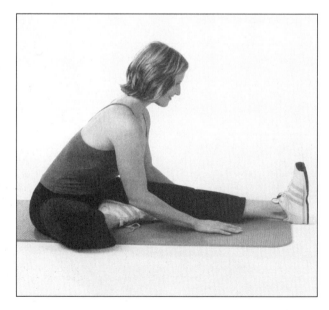

SEATED INNER THIGH STRETCH

Many people have limited flexibility in their inner thighs; take care not to overdo this stretch.

TECHNIQUE AND FORM

1 Sit on the floor or mat with your heels pressed together and your knees out to the side; place your hands around your ankles.

2 As you exhale, press your elbows against your thighs, trying to press your thighs closer to the floor.

3 Hold for 20 to 30 seconds.

TRAINER'S TIPS

Really think about pressing your thighs down against the floor as you execute the stretch.

This is a great stretch to have someone help you out with. Your helper kneels behind you and gently but firmly presses her hands against your thighs, lowering them toward the floor.

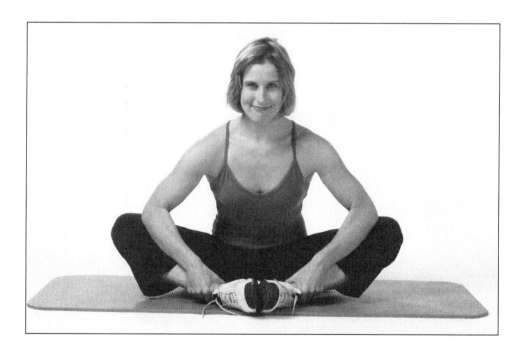

LYING LOWER BACK STRETCH

This super relaxing stretch immediately alleviates strain in your lower back. It simply feels great. Do it whenever you feel your back is tight.

TECHNIQUE AND FORM

1 Lie on your back with your legs extended.

2 Exhale as you bend both legs and pull them in toward your chest.

3 Hold for 20 to 30 seconds.

TRAINER'S TIPS

You may lift your head and upper body a bit to increase the range of this stretch.

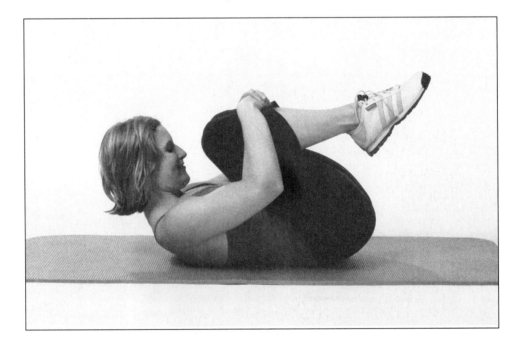

CORE STRETCH

Using the ball provides an increased range for this stretch, which targets your abs and back.

TECHNIQUE AND FORM

1 Sit on a fitness ball; slide down until your lower back is against the ball (as if you are going to perform a crunch on the ball).

2 Slowly walk your feet in close to the ball; at the same time bend backward until your midsection is arched around the ball. Your head and legs with be on opposite sides of the ball.

3 Breathe and hold for 20 to 30 seconds.

TRAINER'S TIPS

 Relax into this stretch. Don't be nervous about bending back; you will not fall.

 To come out of the stretch, slowly walk your feet away from the ball as you lift your upper body.

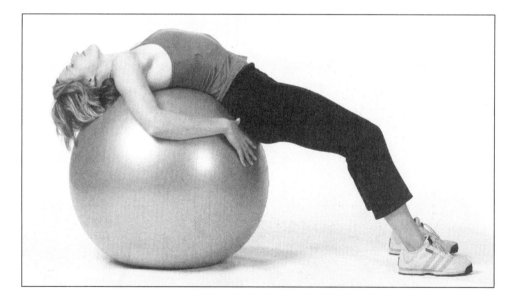

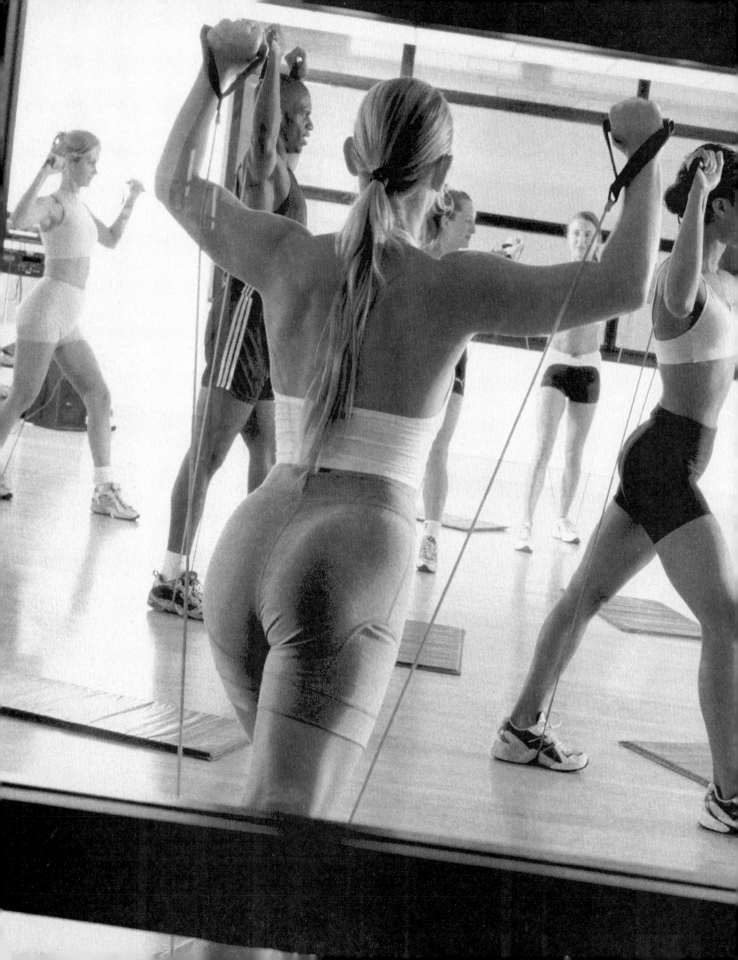

Chapter 4
Glutes and Quads

The basic exercises for the gluteus muscles (butt) and quadriceps (thighs) include the squat, lunge, and leg press. All work both the butt and thigh muscle groups; the degree to which you emphasize the glutes over the quads in a given exercise often is determined by your leg positioning, and the emphasis you give to the positive (lifting) and negative (lowering) phases of each repetition.

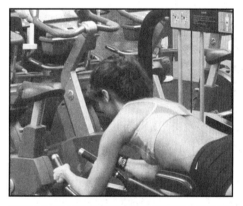

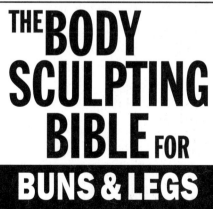

THE BODY SCULPTING BIBLE FOR BUNS & LEGS

4

DUMBBELL SQUAT

The squat is one of the most effective and efficient exercises you can do for many of the muscles in the legs, including your glutes, hamstrings, and quadriceps. Not only do squats help develop shapely legs, but they involve recruitment of your core muscles and enhance balance and stability as well.

TECHNIQUE AND FORM

1 Stand in neutral position, with your feet about hip-width apart; hold a dumbbell in each hand.

2 Bend at your knees and press your hips out behind you.

3 Lower into the squat position (coming no lower than the point where your thighs are parallel to the floor—any lower and you risk knee injury).

4 Exhale, pull your abdominals in and slowly come up to the standing position.

5 Inhale and lower back to the squat position.

6 Repeat for the desired number of repetitions.

TRAINER'S TIPS

✪ Keep your body weight centered over your heels rather than your toes; this will help you to be in the right position when you squat down.

✪ Keep your knees in line with your toes.

DUMBBELL SQUAT

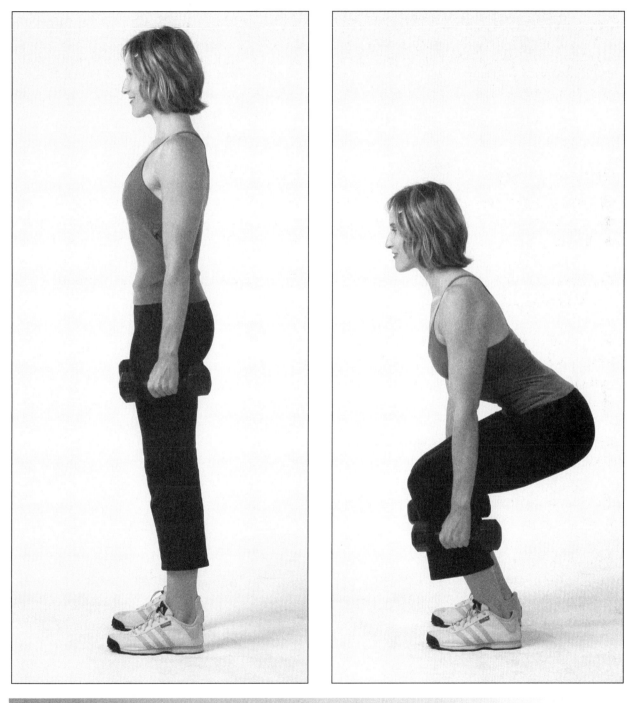

MULTI-DIRECTIONAL LUNGES

This variation of the traditional lunge involves quick changes in direction, and is especially good for improving stability and balance as well as defining your thighs and butt. Note that each repetition of this exercise really involves three lunges, each performed at a different angle.

TECHNIQUE AND FORM

1 Stand in neutral position, with your legs about shoulder-width apart.

2 Step forward with you right leg; keep your head, shoulders, and hips in alignment.

3 Bend both legs so that your right knee makes a 90-degree angle with the floor and left knee comes close to the floor.

4 Lift up and return to the starting position (as you lift make sure you push off with the right foot).

5 Pivot 45 degrees to your right and lunge again with the right leg, returning to the start position after completing the lunge.

6 For the third lunge, once again face forward but this time lunge back with your right leg.

7 Repeat all three lunges with the left leg.

8 Repeat for the desired number of repetitions.

TRAINER'S TIPS

✪ Concentrate on keeping your back straight throughout the lunge; avoid leaning forward.

✪ Make sure you bend your back leg so that it almost touches the floor—it is far better to perform this exercise slowly in a full range of motion than to rush through it and come down only halfway.

✪ When you pivot to perform the 45-degree lunge make sure that your knee is in line with your toes before you lunge.

MULTI-DIRECTIONAL LUNGES

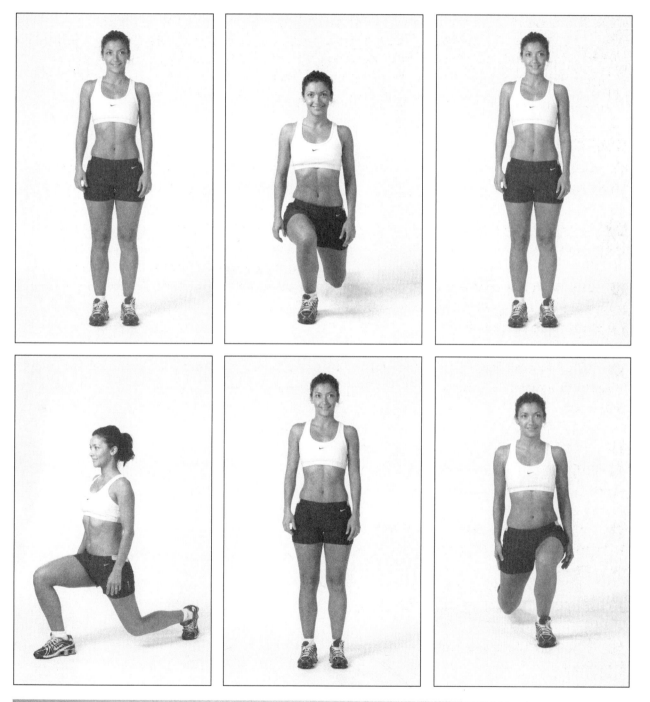

ONE-LEGGED SQUAT

This squat recruits different muscle fibers and accentuates balance and stability.

TECHNIQUE AND FORM

1 Stand in neutral position, with your feet about hip-width apart; hold a dumbbell in each hand.

2 Bend your right leg back so that your right foot is raised from the floor and you are balanced on your left leg.

3 Lower into the squat position.

4 Exhale, pull your abdominals in and slowly come up to the standing position.

5 Inhale and lower back to the squat position.

6 Repeat for the desired number of repetitions.

TRAINER'S TIPS

 Keep your body weight centered over your balancing heel rather than your toes—this will help you to be in the right position when you squat down.

 Keep your knees in line with your toes.

 Because of the additional balance component to this exercise your range of motion will not be as large as in the regular dumbbell squat. Come down only as far as you can while maintaining balance.

ONE-LEGGED SQUAT

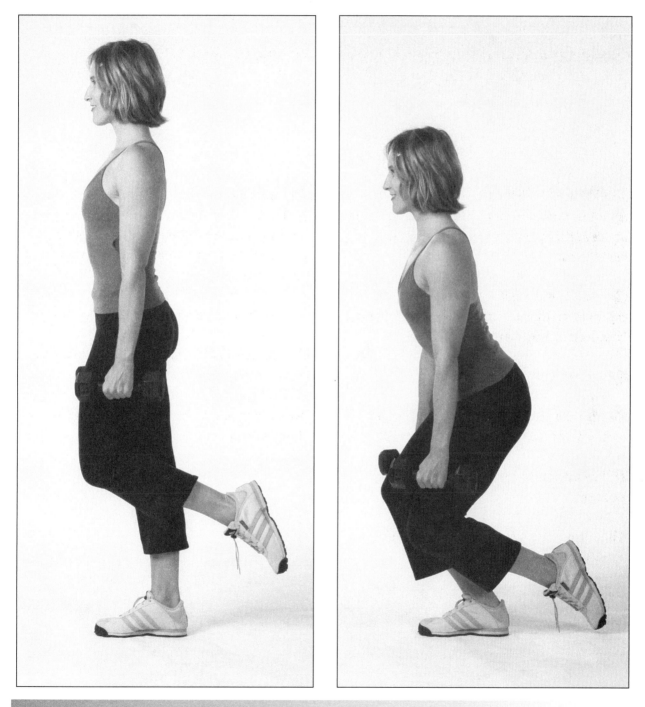

SQUAT WITH BOSU

This variation of the squat is even more challenging. If you don't have access to a BOSU, you can substitute the One-Legged Squat with Fitness Ball, which appears on the following page.

TECHNIQUE AND FORM

1 Stand on the center of the BOSU, with your head up and your abs pulled in and feet about 6 to 8 inches apart. Hold a weight in each hand.

1 Engage your abdominals and lower into a squat position.

2 Exhale and straighten your legs.

3 Inhale and lower into the squat.

4 Repeat for the desired number of repetitions.

TRAINER'S TIPS

 Make sure you are balanced in the center of the ball. As you develop greater kinesthetic awareness and balancing ability, you may be able to perform a squat on one leg.

 It is essential that you keep you chest high and your abs engaged in order to keep your body on the BOSU.

SQUAT WITH BOSU

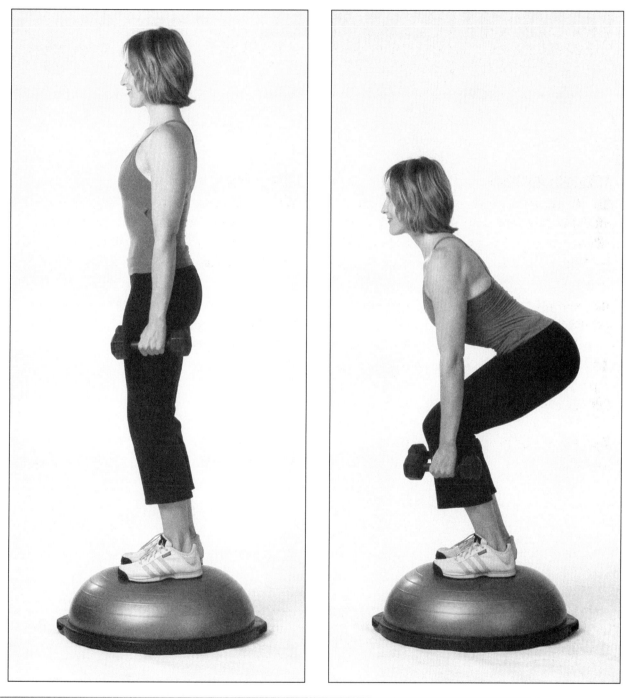

ONE-LEGGED SQUAT WITH FITNESS BALL

Use this version of the squat to increase the balance and stability challenge.

TECHNIQUE AND FORM

1 Stand in front of a wall in neutral position, with your feet shoulder-width apart.

2 Place a fitness ball in between your lower back and the wall.

3 Bend your right leg and hold it in front of you. Lower yourself until your left thigh is almost parallel to the floor.

4 Slowly rise to the starting position.

5 Repeat for the desired number of repetitions.

6 Switch legs.

TRAINER'S TIPS

✪ Pull your navel in toward your spine and the ball in order to stabilize the ball behind you.

✪ This exercise, along with several other fun and challenging fitness ball exercises, can be found in *PowerSculpt for Women* by Paul Frediani (Healthy Living Books, 2005).

ONE-LEGGED SQUAT WITH FITNESS BALL

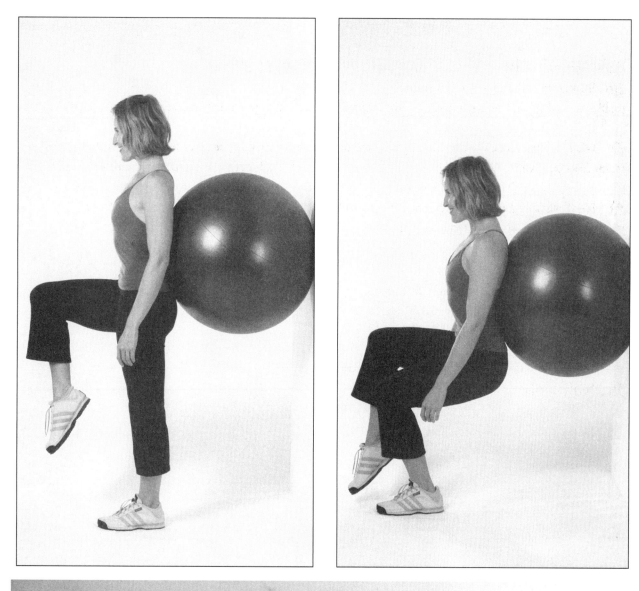

BALL LUNGE

Use a fitness ball to target your butt and thigh muscles a bit differently and to increase the work involved in your stabilizers.

TECHNIQUE AND FORM

1 Stand in front of a fitness ball in neutral position, with your abdominals pulled in and your feet shoulder-width apart. Hold a weight in each hand.

2 Place your right shin on the ball.

3 Bend your left leg as you roll the ball backward with your right foot.

4 Lower your body until your left thigh makes as close to a 90-degree angle with the floor as is possible.

5 As you straighten, roll the ball back to the starting position.

6 Repeat for the desired number of repetitions.

7 Switch sides.

TRAINER'S TIPS

 If you have trouble balancing with the ball, you can place one hand against a wall for support.

BALL LUNGE

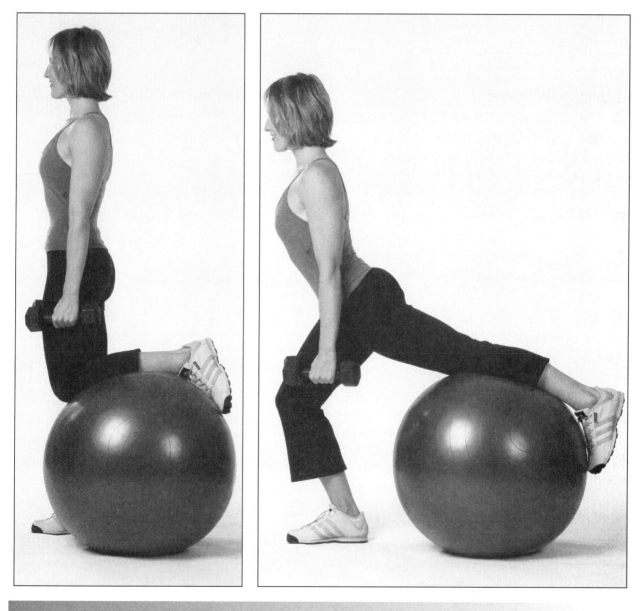

ONE-LEGGED BUTT PRESS WITH BALL

This exercise targets your gluteals, and strengthens your lower back and other core muscles at the same time.

TECHNIQUE AND FORM

1 Sit on top of a fitness ball, your feet shoulder-width apart.

2 Slowly walk your feet forward, so that the ball rolls down your back until it touches your shoulders. Keep your head in line with your spine and keep your butt down. (For additional support, you can also do this exercise resting your head and neck on the ball.)

3 Lift and extend your right leg until it is parallel to the floor; balance and stabilize with your left foot.

4 Press your hips up until they are in line with your knees; squeeze your glutes in the top position before slowly lowering your hips.

5 Repeat for the desired number of repetitions.

6 Switch sides.

TRAINER'S TIPS

You don't need a huge extension for this exercise to be effective; in fact, you should be careful not to hyperextend your back and hip. Concentrate instead on squeezing your gluteal muscles as you lift.

ONE-LEGGED BUTT PRESS WITH BALL

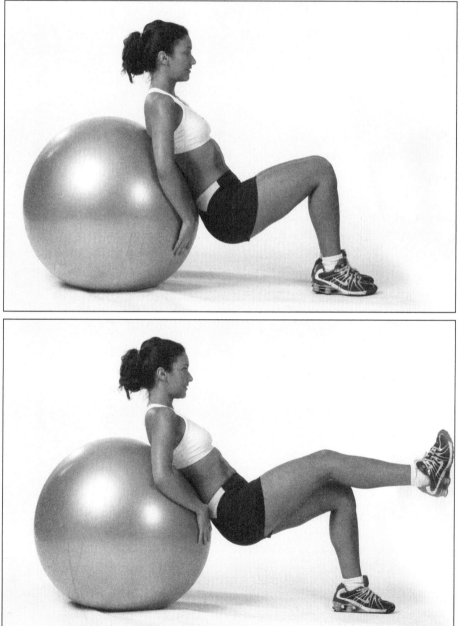

LEG PRESS ON MACHINE

This is a good basic exercise for the legs, albeit not as effective as a dumbbell squat.

FREE WEIGHT ALTERNATIVE: Dumbbell Squat

TECHNIQUE AND FORM

1 Using a leg press machine, sit down and place your legs on the platform directly in front of you at a medium (shoulder-width) foot stance.

2 Lower the safety bars holding the weighted platform in place and press the platform all the way up until your legs are fully extended in front of you (Note: Do not lock your knees). Your torso and the legs should make perfect 90-degree angle. This will be your starting position.

3 As you inhale, slowly lower the platform until your upper and lower legs make a 90-degree angle.

4 Pushing mainly with the toes and using the quadriceps, return to the starting position as you exhale.

5 Repeat for the recommended number of repetitions and be sure to lock the safety pins properly once you are done. You do not want that platform falling on you fully loaded.

TRAINER'S TIPS

To be extra careful, exit the machine after each set by getting your legs out first to one side and then following with your body. We have seen cases in which the safety locks have failed and the whole platform has come tumbling down.

There are other versions of this machine, in which you perform the leg press from a seated or semi-recumbent position. Try to use these types of machines if you have any concerns about manipulating the safety locks.

LEG PRESS ON MACHINE

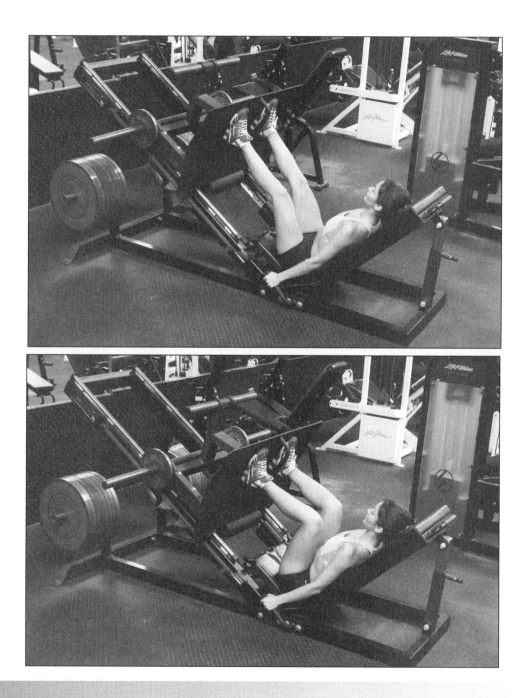

LEG EXTENSION ON MACHINE

This is a great machine for isolating the quadriceps muscles in the fronts of your thighs.

FREE WEIGHT ALTERNATIVE: Multi-Directional Lunges

TECHNIQUE AND FORM

❶ First choose your weight and sit on the machine with your legs under the pad (feet pointed forward) and your hands holding the side bars. This will be your starting position. Note: You will need to adjust the pad so that it falls on top of your lower leg (just above your feet). Also, make sure that your legs form a 90-degree angle between the lower and upper leg. If the angle is less than 90 degrees, the knee is over the toes, which in turn creates undue stress at the knee joint. If the machine is designed that way, either look for another machine or just make sure that when you start executing the exercise you stop going down once you hit the 90-degree angle.

❷ Using your quadriceps, extend your legs to the maximum as you exhale. Ensure that the rest of the body remains stationary on the seat. Pause a second in the contracted position.

❸ Slowly lower the weight back to the original position as you inhale, ensuring that you do not go past the 90-degree angle limit.

❹ Repeat for the desired number of repetitions.

TRAINER'S TIPS

✪ Avoid a fast, jerking motion on the way up; this puts undue stress on the kneecaps.

✪ As stressed in the description above, make sure that your legs form a 90-degree angle between the lower and upper leg.

LEG EXTENSION ON MACHINE

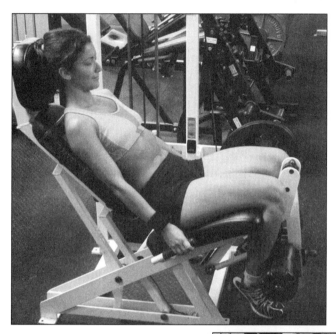

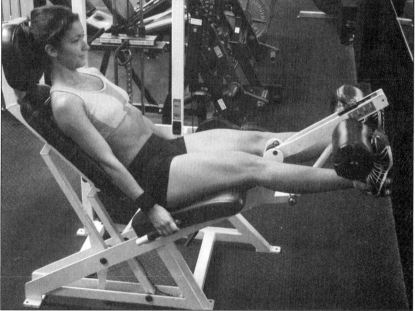

BUTT BLASTER ON MACHINE

This machine hones in on the gluteal muscles by isolating them one leg at a time.

FREE WEIGHT ALTERNATIVE: Dumbbell Squat

TECHNIQUE AND FORM

1 Select the weight with the machine's pins.

2 Get on your hands and knees holding on to the handles.

3 Lift your right leg up behind you, keeping it bent at a 90-degree angle; if the machine has a platform, place the sole of that foot up against the platform. This is your start position.

4 Exhale and press your leg up as you squeeze your gluteal muscles.

5 When you reach the top position, hold for a count or two before lowering to the start position. (This time, however, do not allow the platform to come entirely down because you want to maintain tension in the muscles before you begin the next repetition).

6 Repeat for the desired number of repetitions.

7 Switch sides.

TRAINER'S TIPS

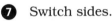 Keep your abdominals pulled in and your back flat as you perform the press. It is important that you keep your back flat like a table throughout the entire range of motion of this exercise to avoid injuring your lower back.

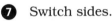 If you feel any pain in your lower back, lighten up on the weight or select a different exercise for the gluetals.

BUTT BLASTER ON MACHINE

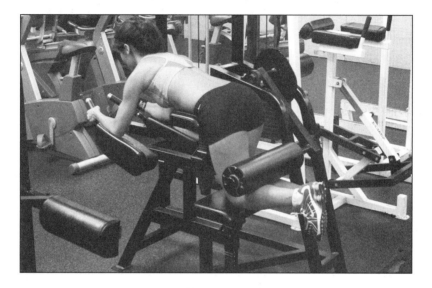

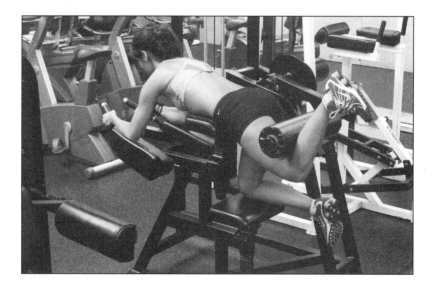

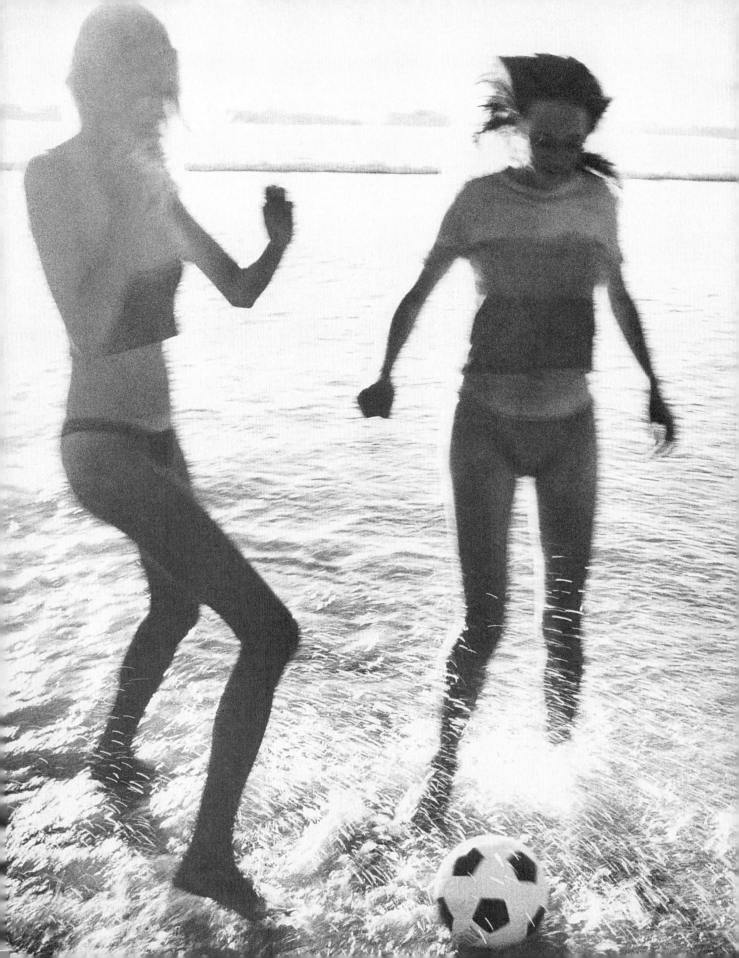

Chapter 5

Inner and Outer Thighs

The inner and outer thighs—frequently problem, flabby areas for women—contain muscles that adduct (move closer to the midline of your body) and abduct (move away from the midline of your body) your legs. This chapter is an all-out attack on these muscles and includes exercises utilizing machines, free weights, the fitness ball, BOSU, and working your body weight against gravity.

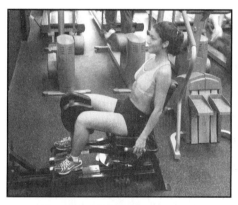

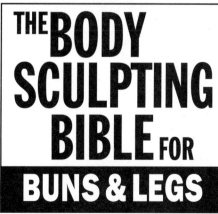

THE **BODY SCULPTING BIBLE** FOR
BUNS & LEGS

SIDE LYING LEG RAISE

This exercise can be performed initially with no resistance before placing a weight on your inner thigh.

TECHNIQUE AND FORM

1 Lie on your side, with your hips straight and knees in alignment. Bend your top leg over your bottom leg so that the inner thigh of the bottom leg faces the ceiling. Your bottom leg remains extended. Your head may rest on the floor or you may prop yourself up on your forearm, whichever position is more comfortable for you. Place a weight on the inner high of your bottom leg.

2 Exhale and lift your bottom leg until you feel tension in the inner thigh muscles. At the top position hold for a second before lowering to the point where your leg is close to but does not touch the floor or mat.

3 Repeat for the desired number of repetitions.

4 Switch sides.

TRAINER'S TIPS

Make sure that your inner thigh is facing the ceiling throughout this exercise. This will ensure maximal recruitment of your adductor muscles.

This exercise requires a lot of concentration; focus on lifting from your inner thigh and not from your lower leg.

SIDE LYING LEG RAISE

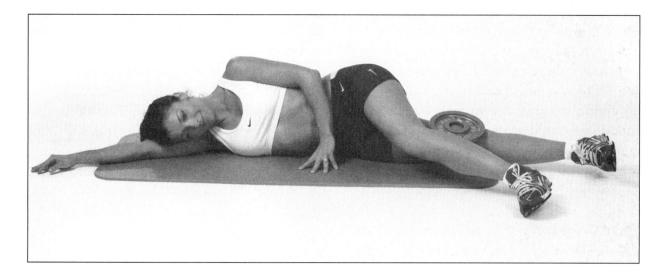

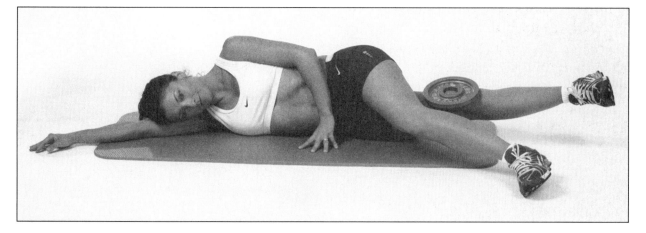

LATERAL LUNGE

This variation of the lunge changes the angle so that your inner thighs have to work harder.

TECHNIQUE AND FORM

1 Stand in neutral position with a weight in each hand and your legs about shoulder-width apart. This is your starting position.

2 Rotate your right hip to take a wide step to the side; your right knee should be in line with the toes of your right foot, which should be facing right. Your left leg remains stationary, with toes facing front.

3 Exhale and lunge to the right, concentrating on pressing your right inner thigh back as you bend your right knee.

4 Come up from the lunge, returning to the starting position, with both legs facing front.

5 Repeat, this time lunging to the left side.

6 Repeat for the desired number of repetitions.

TRAINER'S TIPS

✪ When you lunge, make sure that you do not bend your knee so far that it extends beyond your toes as this position may injure your knee.

✪ Make sure your chest and shoulders remain facing front for the duration of this exercise.

✪ Really think about engaging the muscles in the inner thigh when you perform the lunge.

LATERAL LUNGE

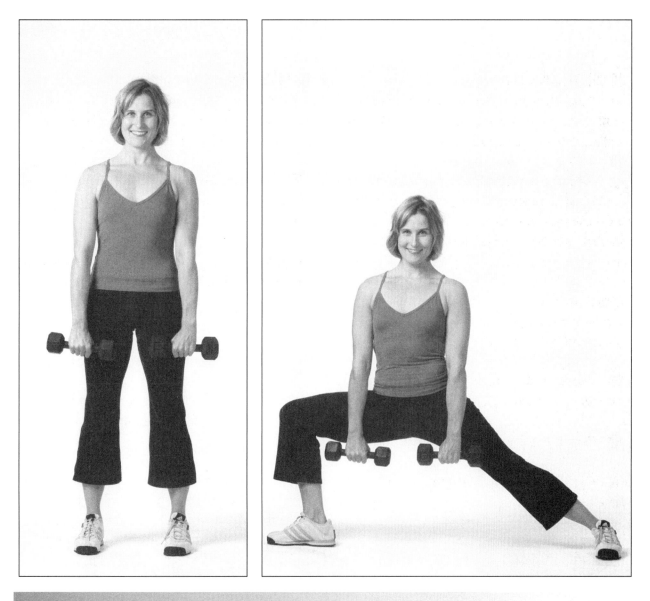

LATERAL LUNGE ONTO BOSU OR STEP

This variation of the lateral lunge adds a balance component with the inclusion of the BOSU or step bench.

TECHNIQUE AND FORM

1 Stand in neutral position with a weight in each hand and your legs about shoulder-width apart. This is your starting position.

2 Rotate your right hip to take a wide step on to the center of the BOSU; your right knee should be in line with the toes of your right foot, which should be facing right. Your left leg remains stationary, with toes facing front.

3 Exhale and lunge to the right, concentrating on pressing your right inner thighs back as you bend your right knee.

4 Come up from the lunge, returning to the starting position—off the BOSU—with both legs facing front.

5 Repeat for the desired number of repetitions

6 Switch sides.

TRAINER'S TIPS

✪ Engage your abdominals as you lunge to the side; this will help you to maintain your balance and stability on the BOSU.

✪ You may need to use lighter weight than you would for the lateral lunge without the BOSU—at least until you've developed greater stability.

✪ When you lunge, make sure that you do not bend your knee so far that it extends beyond your toes as this position may injure your knee.

✪ Make sure your chest and shoulders remain facing front for the duration of this exercise.

✪ Really think about engaging the muscles in the inner thigh when you perform the lunge.

✪ If you do not have a BOSU, you can perform this exercise lunging on to a bench instead. While you will not get as many balance benefits using the bench, you will hit the muscles at different angles, and there is some stability work involved.

LATERAL LUNGE ONTO BOSU OR STEP

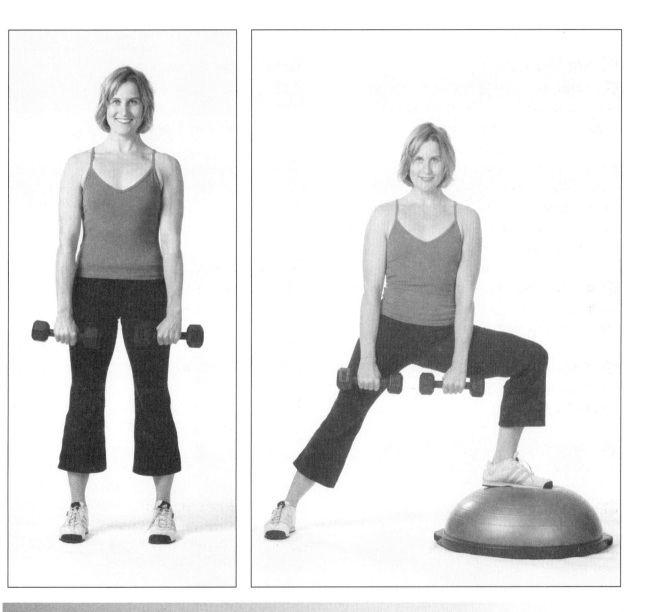

ADDUCTOR ON MACHINE

The Adductor on Machine is a great isolator for the inner thigh muscle group. Make sure you do not set the machine to too wide a position.

FREE WEIGHT ALTERNATIVE: Side Lying Leg Raise

TECHNIQUE AND FORM

1 Sit on the machine with your back straight and head in line with your spine. Position the pads on either side so that they rest against your inner thighs. Select your weight.

2 Use the handles at the sides of the machine to adjust the width (range of motion) between your legs. In general, the width should cause you to feel some tension in your inner thighs in the start position but not place great strain on them.

3 Exhale as you bring your legs toward each other, maintaining tension throughout the exercise.

4 Inhale as you separate your legs and return to the starting position.

5 Repeat for the desired number of repetitions.

TRAINER'S TIPS

If you have to exert a lot of effort to bring your legs together, or start to compensate by using your back or torso, you need to either lighten up on the weight or reduce the range of motion (width between the pads).

To increase the challenge of this exercise, sit straight up without resting your back against the back pad as you perform your reps.

ADDUCTOR ON MACHINE

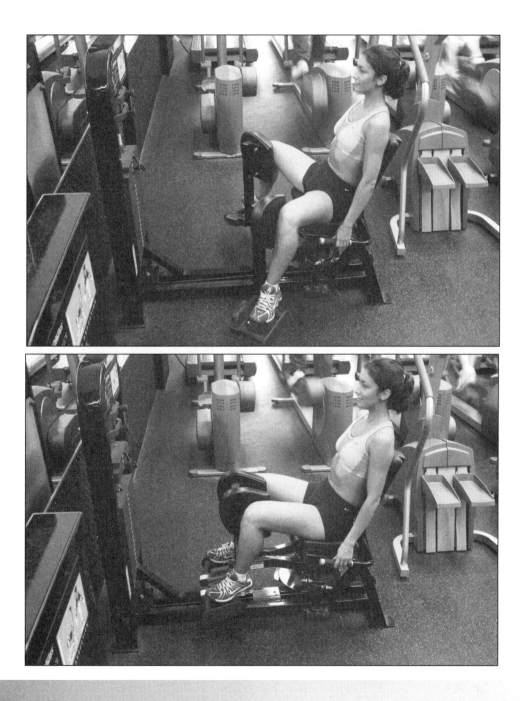

CABLE LEG RAISE

The cable leg raise is a machine version of the side lying leg raise. Some machines (such as the Free Motion) provide resistance on both the contraction and extension phases of the repetition.

FREE WEIGHT ALTERNATIVE: Lateral Lunge

TECHNIQUE AND FORM

1 Set the pin to the desired resistance and attach the foot straps to the cables (The levers of the machine should be in a down position close to the floor).

2 Place the foot strap around the ankle of your right leg as you hold on to the cable machine base with your right arm for support.

3 Exhale and cross your right leg in front of your left leg so that the inner thigh of your right leg is working to lift the leg. Go as high as you need to feel tension in the muscles. Hold for a second.

4 Slowly return to the start position as you exhale (do not come fully down to the floor).

5 Repeat for the desired number of repetitions.

6 Switch sides.

TRAINER'S TIPS

Keep your back straight and your body in good postural alignment throughout the exercise. Engaging your abdominals is essential.

Once you complete one repetition, do not rest before performing the next—it is important that you maintain tension consistently for an entire set.

CABLE LEG RAISE

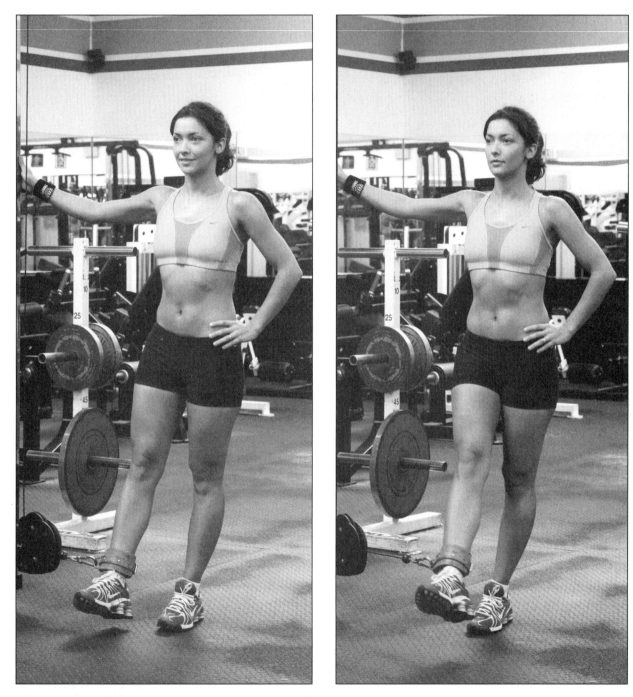

WIDE STANCE SQUAT

The wide stance squat is similar to the dumbbell squat, but your legs are wider apart, placing greater emphasis on your inner quads and inner thighs.

TECHNIQUE AND FORM

1 Stand in neutral position, with your feet one and a half times wider than your shoulders and your toes pointed to the side; hold a dumbbell in each hand.

2 Bend at your knees and press your hips out behind you.

3 Inhale as you lower into the squat position (coming no lower than the point where your thighs are parallel to the floor—any lower and you risk knee injury).

4 Exhale, pull your abdominals in and slowly come up to the standing position.

5 Inhale and lower back down to the squat position.

6 Repeat for the desired number of repetitions.

TRAINER'S TIPS

Be careful not too take too wide a stance, as this may injure your inner thighs or knees.

Keep your back straight and your head up (in line with your spine) throughout the squat.

WIDE STANCE SQUAT

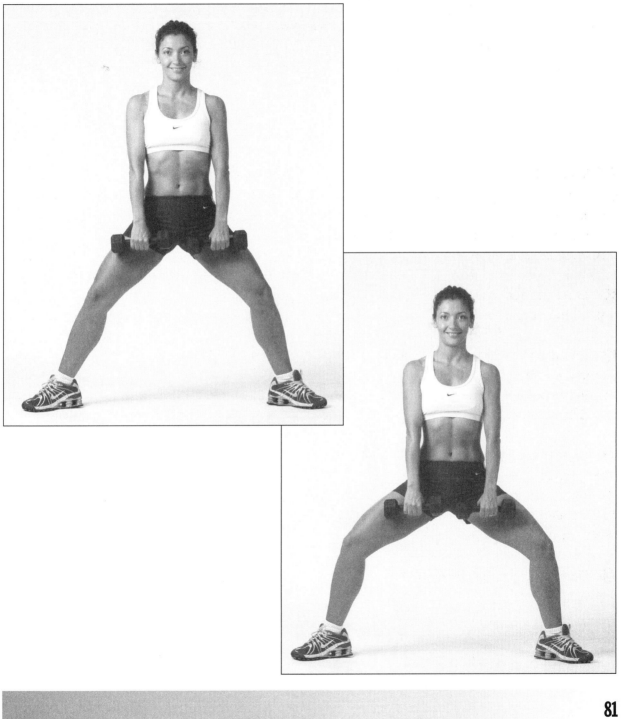

BALL EXTENSION

With this ball exercise you work the fronts of your thighs, your inner thighs, and your core.

TECHNIQUE AND FORM

1 Lie on your back on a mat with your legs raised, your knees bent, and the ball held with the lower parts of your legs. (You should feel as if you are grabbing the ball with your lower legs).

2 As you exhale, slowly extend your legs to the ceiling until they are almost locked.

3 Hold for a second at the top position and squeeze the ball hard before slowly lowering to the start position.

4 Repeat for the desired number of repetitions.

TRAINER'S TIPS

Keep your lower back pressed against the mat or floor at all times. ONLY your legs are moving during this exercise.

To maximize inner thigh work, concentrate on using your leg muscles to squeeze in toward the ball as your straighten and bend your legs. Maintain tension in the inner thighs throughout the exercise.

BALL EXTENSION

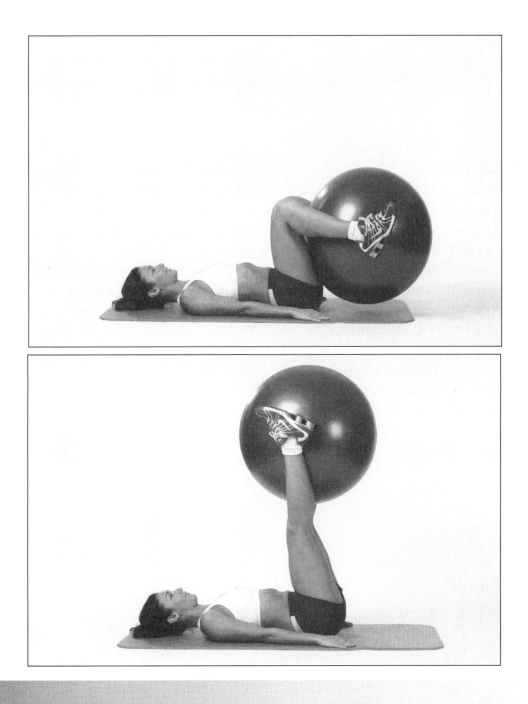

SIDE LYING OUTER THIGH RAISE

This exercise can be performed initially with no resistance, before placing a weight on your outer thigh.

TECHNIQUE AND FORM

1 Lie on your side, with your hips and knees in alignment, and your bottom leg bent at the knee. Your head may rest on the floor or you may prop yourself up on your forearm, whichever position is more comfortable for you. Place a weight on the outer thigh of your top leg.

2 Exhale and lift your top leg until you feel tension in the outer thigh muscles. At the top position hold for a second before lowering to the point where your top leg comes close to but does not touch your bottom leg.

3 Repeat for the desired number of repetitions.

4 Switch sides.

TRAINER'S TIPS

 Make sure that your outer thigh is facing the ceiling throughout this exercise. This will ensure maximal recruitment of your abductor muscles.

SIDE LYING OUTER THIGH RAISE

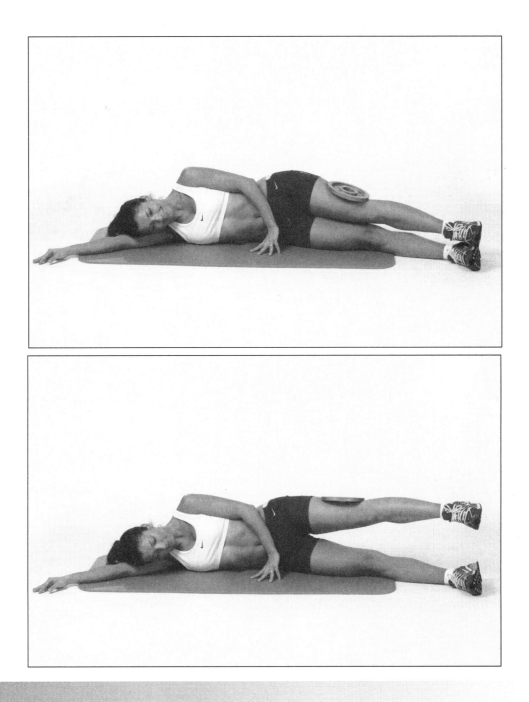

CABLE LEG RAISE FOR OUTER THIGH

The cable leg raise is a machine version of the standing or lying leg raise.

FREE WEIGHT ALTERNATIVE: Squat with Abduction

TECHNIQUE AND FORM

1 Set the pin to the desired resistance and attach the foot straps to the cables (The levers of the machine should be in a down position close to the floor).

2 Place the foot strap around the ankle of the outer leg as you hold on to the cable machine base with for support.

3 Exhale and extend your leg out to the side, engaging your outer thigh muscles. Go as high as you need to feel tension in the muscles. Hold for a second.

4 Slowly return to the start position as you exhale (do not come fully down to the floor).

5 Repeat for the desired number of repetitions.

6 Switch sides.

TRAINER'S TIPS

✪ Keep your back straight and your body in good postural alignment throughout the exercise. Engaging your abdominals is essential.

✪ One you complete one repetition, do not rest before performing the next—it is important that you maintain tension consistently for an entire set.

CABLE LEG RAISE FOR OUTER THIGH

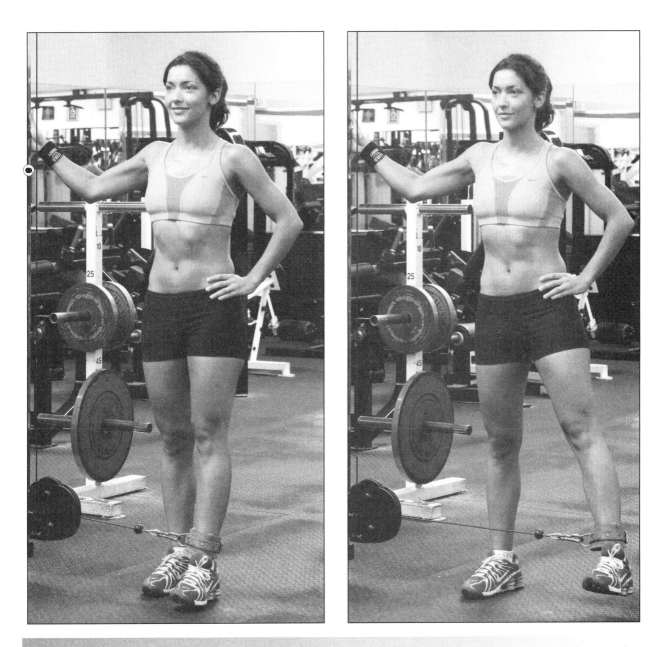

SIDE LEG KICK

This exercise works balance and stability in addition to toning your outer thighs. Begin with no resistance and add it only in small increments (a couple of pounds) if you find you need the extra weight. You may need a body bar or a broom to help you balance.

TECHNIQUE AND FORM

1 Stand in neutral position. Lightly rest your right hand on a body bar or broom (which should be positioned just to the right of your right foot) to help you balance, if needed.

2 If you are using additional resistance, hold the light weight on your outer thigh, just below your left hip.

3 Exhale and lift your left leg out to the side, coming up as far as you need to feel tension in your outer thigh muscles. To maintain balance as you do this, press your right foot firmly into the floor, engage your abdominals, and hold your chest high.

4 Hold the top position for a second before returning the leg back down.

5 Repeat for the desired number of repetitions before switching to the other leg.

TRAINER'S TIPS

Do not lift your leg too high. If you feel pain instead of a tensing of the muscles, you are lifting too high.

Really think about the muscles you are working during this exercise.

Do not bear down on the bar or broom—you are only using it to give you a bit of balance support.

SIDE LEG KICK

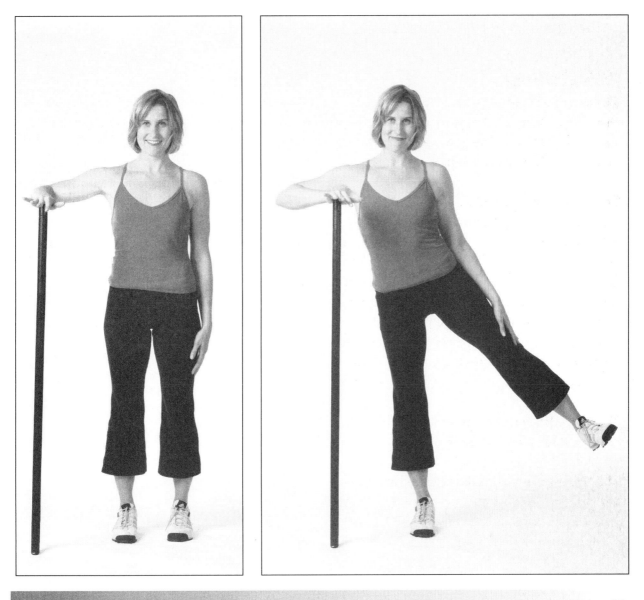

SQUAT WITH ABDUCTION

Control is essential in this great exercise for the gluteals, outer thighs, and stabilizers. Never kick wildly.

TECHNIQUE AND FORM

1 Stand straight, with your knees slightly bent and a slight curve to your spine, and your feet approximately shoulder-width apart. Hold a dumbbell in each hand; keep your arms down by your sides.

2 Inhale and lower into the squat position with your knees bent, your hips pressed out behind you, and your thighs no lower than parallel to the floor.

3 Exhale as you straighten your legs; once they are almost straight press your left leg out to the side.

4 As you bring your left leg down, immediately perform a squat.

5 Repeat; this time pressing your right leg out to the side as you come out of the squat.

6 Repeat the sequence for desired number of repetitions.

TRAINER'S TIPS

Think about PRESSING your leg rather than kicking it—this will help you to use less momentum and more muscle.

You don't have to lift your leg up high to get benefits from this exercise: lift high enough so that you feel a tightening in your outer thighs, but never any sharp pain.

To increase intensity of this exercise you can perform side arm raises with dumbbells as you come out of the squat.

SQUAT WITH ABDUCTION

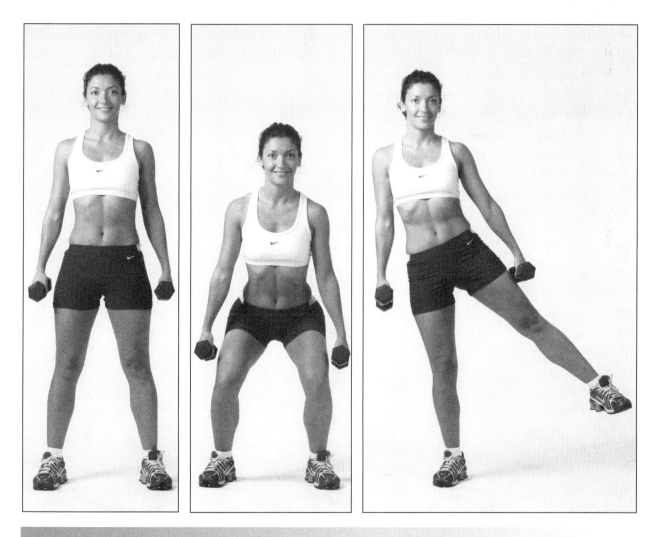

ABDUCTOR ON MACHINE

The Abductor on Machine is a great isolator for the outer thigh muscle group.

FREE WEIGHT ALTERNATIVE: Side Lying Outer Thigh Leg Raise

TECHNIQUE AND FORM

1 Sit on the machine with your back straight and head in line with your spine. Use the handles at the sides of the machine to bring your legs to a point where they are nearly touching—this is your start position. Position the pads on either side so that they rest against your outer thighs.

2 Exhale as you separate your legs, maintaining tension throughout the exercise.

3 Inhale as you bring your legs closer together, returning to the starting position.

4 Repeat for the desired number of repetitions.

TRAINER'S TIPS

✪ To increase the challenge of this exercise, sit straight up without resting your back against the back pad as you perform your reps.

ABDUCTOR ON MACHINE

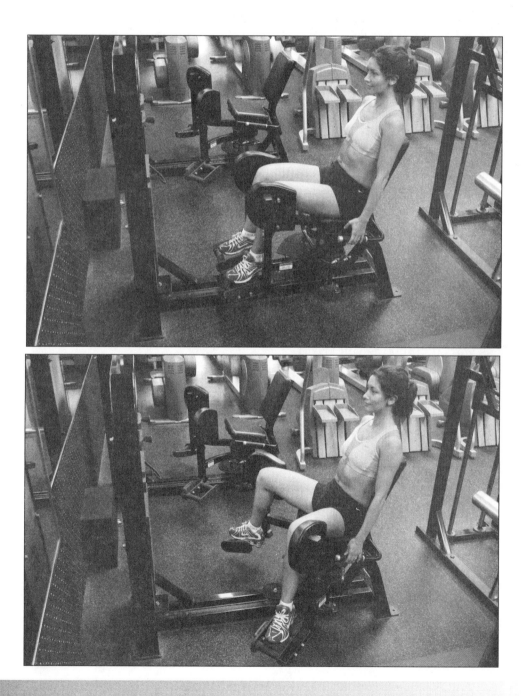

BALL ABDUCTION

Here's another great fitness ball exercise; this one works the outer thighs.

TECHNIQUE AND FORM

1 Lie on your left side on a ball. Place your left hand on the floor for support. Your legs should be stacked.

2 Extend your right leg in front at a 45-degree angle.

3 Keeping your foot flexed, lift and lower the leg (exhale as you lift, inhale as you lower).

TRAINER'S TIPS

Make sure you are pulling your abs in tight throughout this exercise.

Keeping the foot of your working leg flexed with toes pointing down will home in on the buttocks as well as the outer thighs.

BALL ABDUCTION

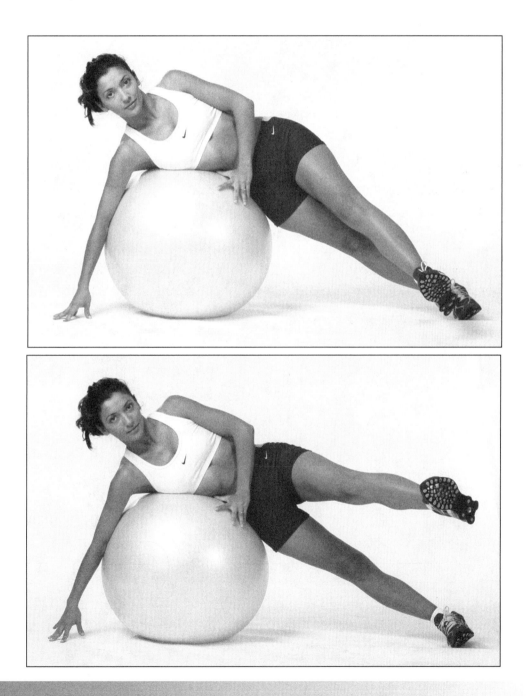

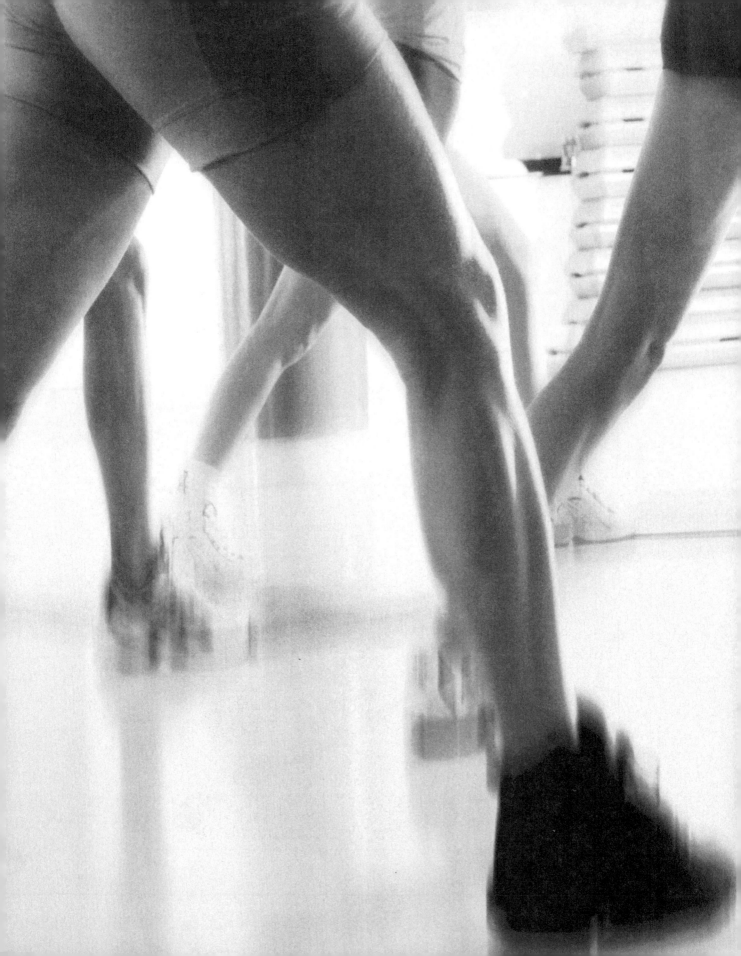

Chapter 6

Hamstrings and Calves

In general, the hamstring muscles in the backs of the legs (also known as the biceps femoris) are very tight. This is especially true for women who engage in high-impact cardio activity such as running and jogging. For this reason, it is essential that you make sure to perform the hamstring stretches described in the stretch chapter whenever you train this muscle group.

The calves take a bit of time to respond to training, and for optimal results you need to train them at a variety of angles. However, the time you take to develop your calves is time well spent: they are a particularly eye-catching part of your legs and well-defined calves look great in heels or flats.

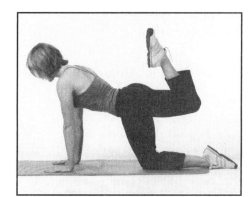

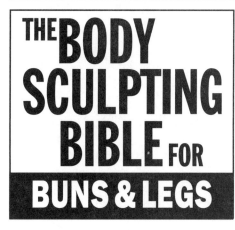

THE BODY SCULPTING BIBLE FOR BUNS & LEGS

CURL ON ALL FOURS

While you do not use any weights for this exercise, it is quite an effective anti-gravity toner for the back of your legs.

TECHNIQUE AND FORM

1. Begin on all fours (hands on the floor) with your back flat and your head in line with your spine. Your elbows should be directly beneath your shoulders and your knees should be directly beneath your hips.

2. Lift your right leg (keeping it bent) until your knee is hip-high.

3. Extend your right leg, straightening it out behind you. This is the starting position.

4. Exhale and curl your right heel in toward your butt for two counts.

5. Inhale and extend your leg back out to the starting position.

6. Repeat for the desired number of repetitions.

7. Switch sides.

TRAINER'S TIPS

- As you perform the exercise it is essential to keep your body balanced over your center of mass (you do not want to lean to one side). To do this, engage your abdominals and concentrate on righting your body if you feel it tilt.

- To increase the tension in this exercise you may use ankle weights.

- As you curl your leg you must use a lot of mental focus and concentration. Think about contracting your hamstrings as hard as you can.

- A variation of this exercise involves first pressing your bent leg up and squeezing the buttocks hard, before performing the curl. (This variation involves some stimulation of the gluteal muscles in your butt).

CURL ON ALL FOURS

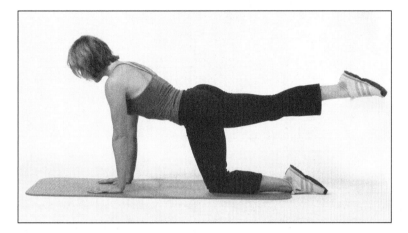

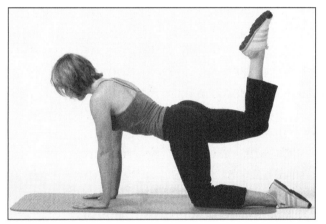

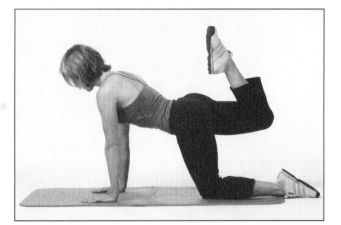

LYING HAMSTRING CURL ON MACHINE

This is a good isolation machine exercise for the hamstrings.

FREE WEIGHT ALTERNATIVE: Curl on All Fours

TECHNIQUE AND FORM

1 Adjust the machine lever to fit your height and lie face down on the leg Curl on Machine (preferably one where the pad is angled instead of flat since an angled position is more favorable for hamstring recruitment) with the pad of the lever positioned on the backs of your legs (just a few inches under the calves).

2 Keeping your torso flat on the bench, be sure your legs are fully stretched and grab the side handles of the machine. Your toes should be straight. This is your starting position.

3 As you exhale, curl your legs as far as possible without lifting your upper legs or hip. Once you hit the fully contracted position, hold for a second.

4 As you inhale, bring the legs back to the initial position.

5 Repeat for the desired number of repetitions.

TRAINER'S TIPS

✖ Never use so much weight that you start to swing or jerk, as you can risk both lower back injury and a hamstring tear.

✖ Try not to rest in between repetitions; as soon as your legs return to the starting position you begin the next curl.

LYING HAMSTRING CURL ON MACHINE

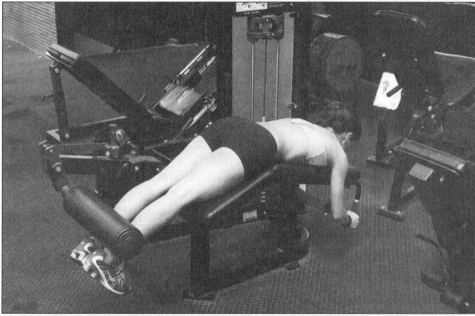

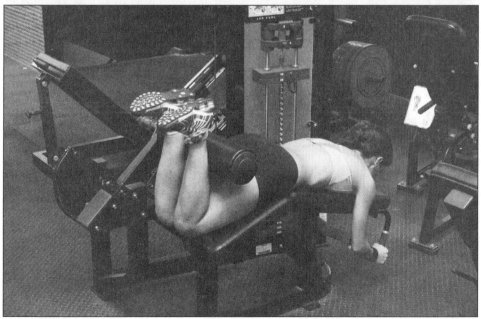

HAMSTRING CURL ON THE BALL

A great hamstring toner that you do with a fitness ball. You will really feel these immediately and, because these exercises require balance and coordination, you will be working on those areas as well!

TECHNIQUE AND FORM

1 Lie on your back on a mat, with your lower legs on the fitness ball. Your hands are straight out to your sides.

2 Lift your buttocks and hips so that you are balancing with your midback muscles and your body forms a straight line from your knees to your shoulders. This is your starting position.

3 Slowly bend your knees as you pull your heels in toward your buttocks, rolling the ball close to your butt.

4 Hold for a second before slowly returning to the start position and continuing, without rest, with the next repetition.

5 Repeat for the desired number of repetitions.

TRAINER'S TIPS

✪ You need to keep the ball steady—it should not roll around under your legs. If you are having difficulty, you can practice just holding the raised position for several seconds. Another modification is to not lift your body so high—keep more of your back in contact with the mat.

✪ To increase the balance challenge, change the position of your arms. Try crossing them over your chest or keeping them down by your sides!

✪ If you have neck problems, you should not perform this exercise.

HAMSTRING CURL ON THE BALL

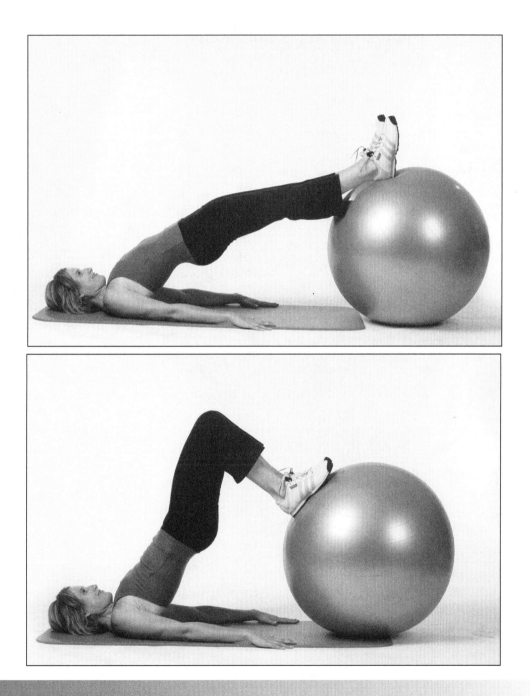

STANDING HAMSTRING CURL

This version of the hamstring curl isolates the hamstring muscles and, because you are working one leg at a time, helps you to address any imbalances you may have in your legs.

TECHNIQUE AND FORM

1 Stand next to the lever arm of the machine, so that it is to the right of your leg.

2 Hook your right heel under the roller pad. (Depending on the machine you use, you will either be able to kneel upon a knee rest with your left leg, or stand with your left leg on a platform.)

3 Keeping your upper leg (from the knee to the hip) in place, exhale and curl your right leg up as high as it can go.

4 At the top of the movement, squeeze the hamstring muscles hard and hold for one to two seconds.

5 Return to the bottom in a controlled motion.

6 Perform desired number of reps for one leg, then switch to the other.

TRAINER'S TIPS

Be sure that you use muscular contraction and not momentum to help you to curl your leg (If you find you are arching your back or using your shoulders to help you to contract, chances are you are using momentum. If this is the case, you may also need to reduce the weight.)

STANDING HAMSTRING CURL

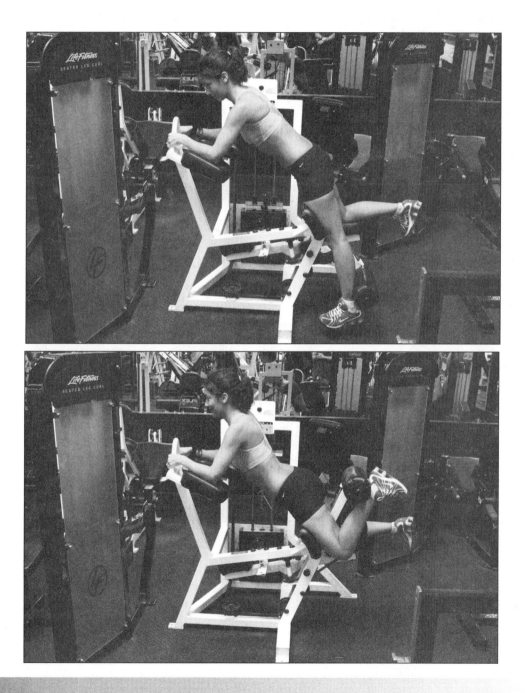

SEATED LEG CURL

Here's a great leg curl machine, especially for those of you with any lower back problems—the back pad provides support for your lumbar spine.

TECHNIQUE AND FORM

1 Sit on the machine with the backs of your legs against the pad; your knees should be aligned with the axis of rotation of the machine.

2 Keeping the tops of your legs (from your hips to your knees) stationary, bend your knees, curling your legs as far as they can go.

3 Squeeze your hamstring muscles hard and hold for a second or two before slowly returning to the starting position.

4 Repeat for the desired number of repetitions.

TRAINER'S TIPS

✪ To help alleviate any pressure on your back, make sure you keep your back straight throughout this exercise.

✪ While you may hold on to the handles at the sides of the machine to keep your body in position, make sure you do not squeeze them too hard—this will divert focus from the hamstrings.

SEATED LEG CURL

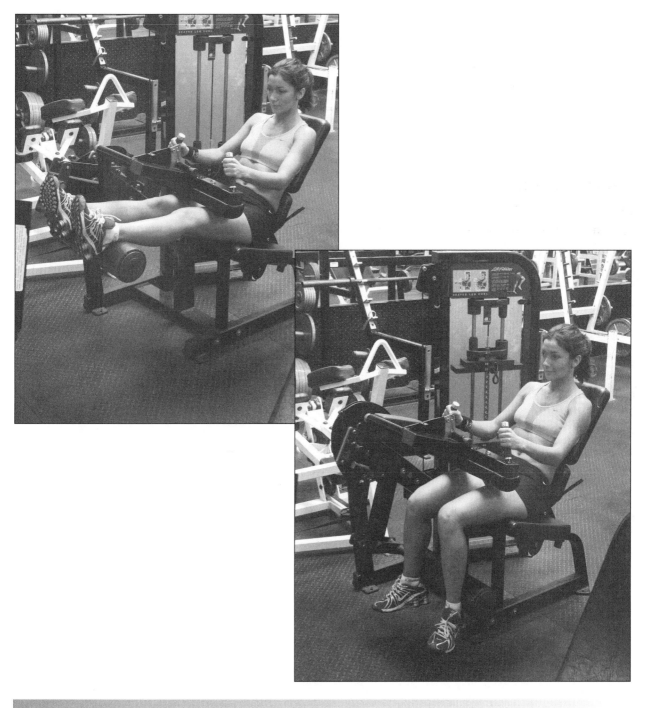

DEADLIFT

This exercise targets both the hamstring muscles at the back of your legs and your lower back muscles. However, this exercise is contraindicated if you suffer from lower back injury because it may strain an already injured back.

TECHNIQUE AND FORM

1 Stand in neutral position, with a weight in each hand, your feet shoulder-width apart, pointing straight ahead, and your legs locked.

2 Bend from your waist, keeping your legs locked out or slightly bent and your arms hanging down in front of your thighs (your palms turned toward your body).

3 Look straight ahead as you bend over. Lower until your upper body is parallel to the floor and the dumbbells are below your knees.

4 Slowly straighten to the starting position.

5 Repeat for the desired number of repetitions.

TRAINER'S TIPS

It is essential that you keep your back flat as a table as you lower; pulling your abdominals in and looking straight ahead will help you to maintain proper form.

Use the power of your mind to focus on the hamstrings—think about the backs of your legs as you work them.

To reduce the strain placed on your back you may perform this exercise with your knees slightly bent. (This position is not as effective a hamstring toner, but it will prevent injury).

DEADLIFT

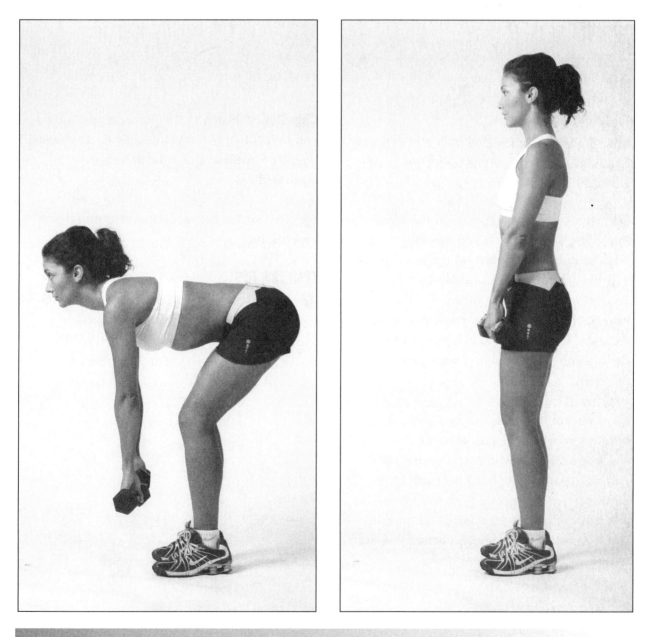

CALF PRESS ON LEG PRESS MACHINE

This movement targets the gastrocnemius muscle, which is the belly of the calf.

FREE WEIGHT ALTERNATIVE: Multi-Directional Calf Raises

TECHNIQUE AND FORM

1 Sit on a leg press machine and place your legs on the platform directly in front of you about six inches apart.

2 Your torso and legs should make a perfect 90-degree angle. Now carefully place your toes and the balls of your feet on the lower portion of the platform with the heels extending off. Your toes can be facing forward, outward, or inward to accentuate different fibers of the calf muscles. Hold on to the handles at the sides of the machine. This will be your starting position.

3 Press on the platform by raising your heels as you breathe out, extending your ankles as far as possible and flexing your calves. Ensure that your knees are kept stationary at all times. Try to keep your legs straight during the exercise. Hold the contracted position for a second before you start to go back down.

4 Slowly return to the starting position as you breathe in by lowering your heels as you bend the ankles until your calves are stretched.

5 Repeat for the recommended number of repetitions.

TRAINER'S TIPS

Make sure that you don't use weight that is too heavy or you will strain your knees.

CALF PRESS ON LEG PRESS MACHINE

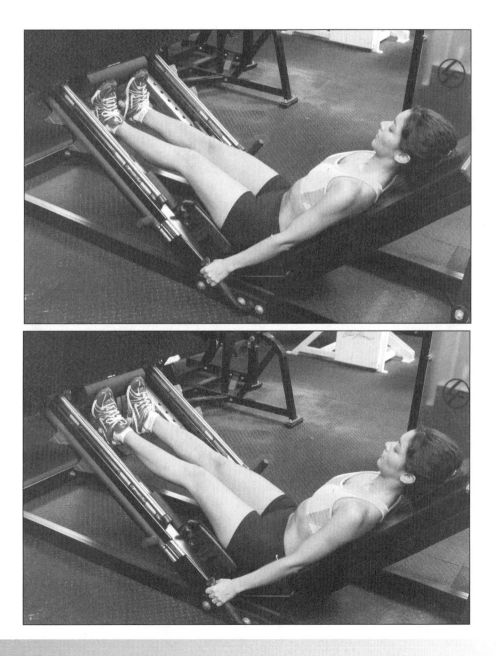

CALF RAISE

This movement also targets the gastrocnemius muscle in the calf.

TECHNIQUE AND FORM

1 Adjust the padded lever of the calf raise machine to fit your height.

2 Place your shoulders under the pads and position your toes facing forward. The balls of your feet should be secured on top of the calf block with the heels extending off it. Push the lever up by extending your hips and knees until your torso is standing erect. The knees should be kept with a slight bend; never locked. Toes should be facing forward. This will be your starting position.

3 Raise your heels as you breathe out by extending your ankles as high as possible and flexing your calves. Keep the knees stationary at all times. There should be no bending at any time. Hold the contracted position for a second before you start to go back down.

4 Go back slowly to the starting position as you breathe in by lowering your heels as you bend the ankles until calves are stretched.

5 Repeat for the recommended number of repetitions.

TRAINER'S TIPS

If you suffer from lower back problems, a better exercise is the calf press because during a standing calf raise the back has to support the weight being lifted.

Maintain a straight, stationary back at all times. Rounding of the back can cause lower back injury.

CALF RAISE

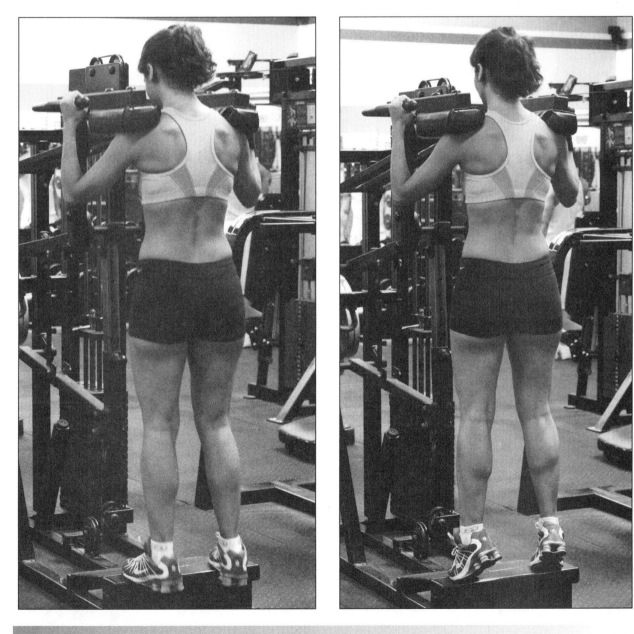

SEATED CALF RAISE

This movement targets the muscle beneath the gastrocnemius. It is a great calf-shaper.

TECHNIQUE AND FORM

❶ Sit on the calf raise machine with your back straight and the padded support fitted snugly on top of your thighs. Position your feet on the platform, with your toes pointing straight ahead. Your toes and the balls of your feet should be on the platform.

❷ Slowly lower your heels toward the floor and bring the calves to a full stretch.

❹ Hold this position for one to two seconds.

❺ Exhale as you push off the balls of your feet and come up to your toes, flexing your calves as hard as you possibly can. Hold for one to two seconds before inhaling and slowly lowering to the stretch position.

❻ Repeat for the desired number of repetitions.

TRAINER'S TIPS

✪ Make sure you keep your head and torso straight and do not lean forward or backward during this exercise.

✪ As you reach the bottom position, control the speed at which your heels drop to the floor.

SEATED CALF RAISE

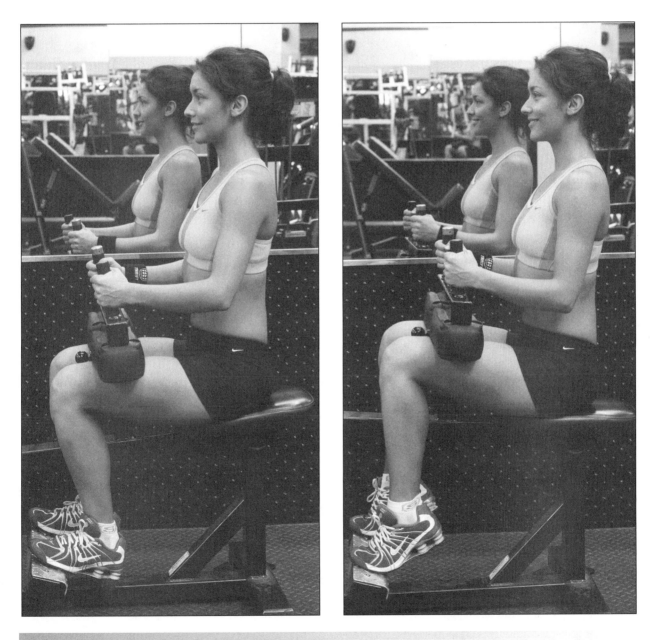

ONE-LEGGED CALF PRESS ON LEG PRESS ON MACHINE

This movement targets the gastrocnemius and soleus muscles of the calves. By performing it one leg at a time, you address any imbalances between your two calves.

TECHNIQUE AND FORM

1 Sit on a leg press machine and place your legs on the platform directly in front of you at a medium (shoulder-width) foot stance.

2 Your torso and legs should make a 90-degree angle. Carefully place the toes and ball of one foot on the lower portion of the platform with the heel extending off. Toes should face forward, outward or inward. This is the starting position.

3 Press on the platform as you breathe out, pressing through your heel. Keep the knee stationary at all times. There should be no bending at any time. Hold the contracted position for a second or two.

4 Slowly return to the starting position as you breathe in and bring your heel back in.

5 Repeat for the recommended number of repetitions on one leg; then switch to the other leg for the recommended number of repetitions.

TRAINER'S TIPS

⊕ Make sure you don't use weight that is too heavy, or you will strain your knees.

ONE-LEGGED CALF PRESS ON LEG PRESS ON MACHINE

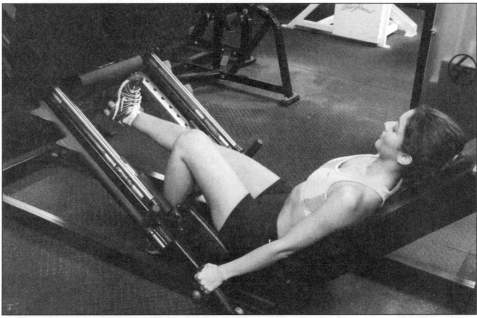

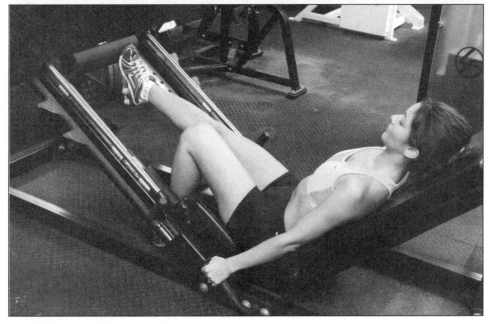

MULTI-DIRECTIONAL CALF RAISES

By performing a series of calf raise at different angles, you target all the muscle fibers involved in providing your calves with sexy definition.

TECHNIQUE AND FORM

1 Stand with your torso upright holding two dumbbells in your hands by your sides. This will be your starting position.

2 With the toes pointing straight, raise the heels off the floor as you exhale by contracting the calves. Hold the top contraction for a second.

3 As you inhale, go back to the starting position by slowly lowering your heels.

4 Repeat for the desired number of repetitions.

5 Perform the next set with toes pointing inward; then with your toes pointing outward.

TRAINER'S TIPS

Notice that for this exercise you won't be able to achieve a full stretch at the bottom unless you are on some kind of platform. The exercise is effective nonetheless.

MULTI-DIRECTIONAL CALF RAISES

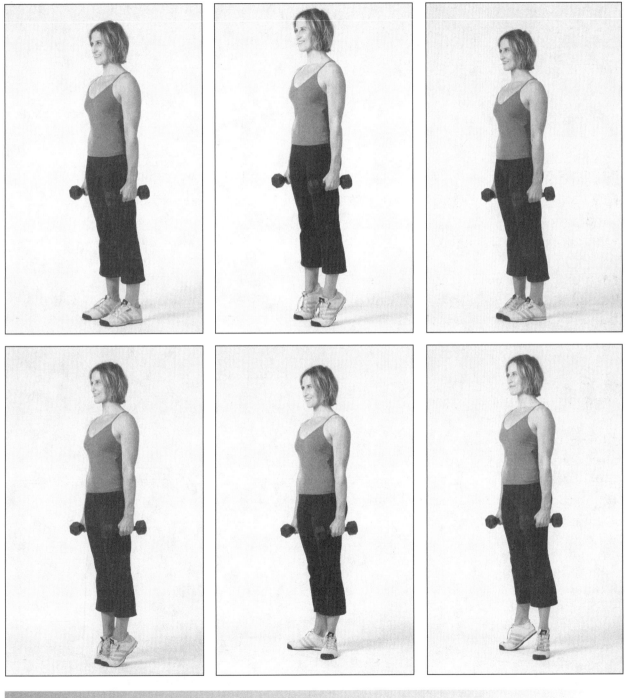

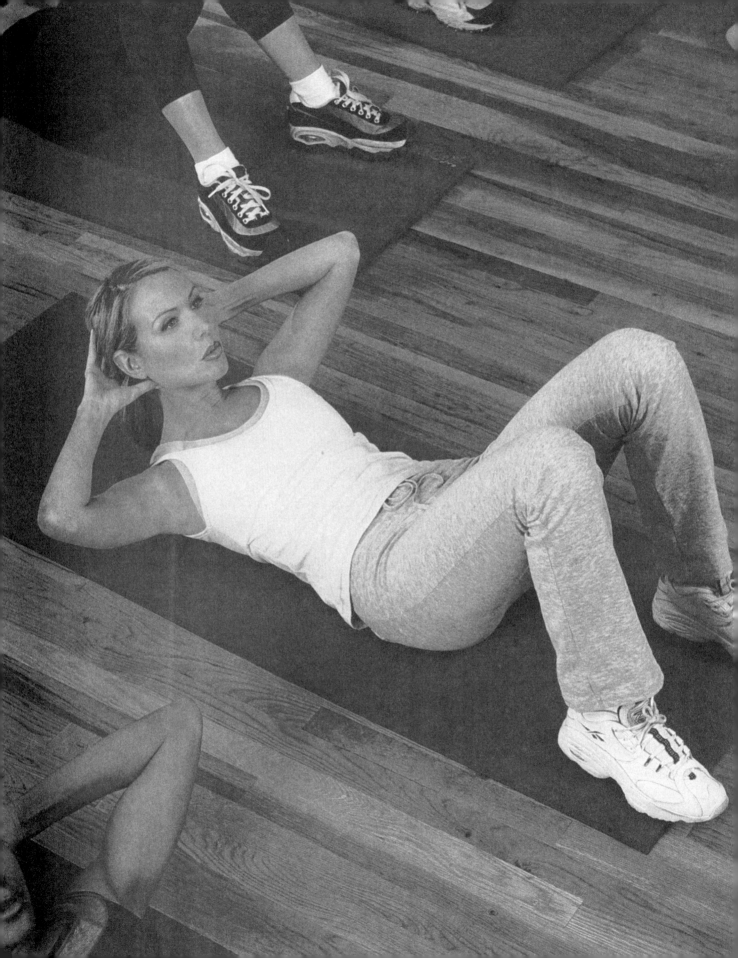

Chapter 7

The Core

Core is a buzzword in the fitness world. What does it really mean? Your core muscles are those at the center or trunk of your body—your abdominals, pelvis, back. All are essential for stabilization and all work together to drive every movement you make. For every free weight exercise you do, you need a strong center to execute the exercise in good form and safely.

The core exercises in this chapter make great use of the fitness ball. Training the core on the ball, a staple now in gyms, which you can easily purchase, is an extremely efficient way to ensure that you target all the muscles of the core. When you perform an exercise on the ball, you recruit muscles in your back, your abdominals, and your pelvis, leaving your center stronger, sculpted, and powerful.

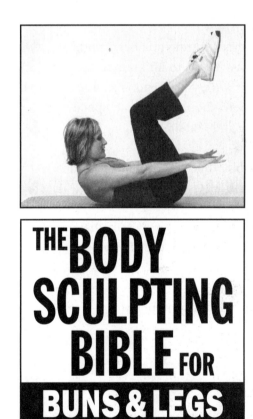

THE BODY SCULPTING BIBLE FOR BUNS & LEGS

7

CRUNCH ON THE BALL

This variation of the traditional abdominal crunch allows for greater range of motion and increased recruitment of core stabilizers.

TECHNIQUE AND FORM

1 Sit on a fitness ball, slide down until your lower back is on the ball. Your shoulders and upper back should be elevated.

2 Cross your arms behind your head and, as you exhale, slowly begin to lift your torso for three counts. Make sure your head is in line with your back (there should be ample space between your chin and chest).

3 At the same time that you lift your chest, you can lift one leg a few inches off the floor.

4 At the top position, hold for a count before lowering your torso and leg to the start position.

5 Repeat for the desired number of repetitions.

TRAINER'S TIPS

For a more intense balance and stabilization exercise, perform with one leg lifted and bent for the entire range of motion.

If you have trouble performing the exercise while lifting one leg, keep both in contact with the floor at all times.

Concentrate on keeping the ball as still as possible while performing the crunch.

If you do not have a ball, perform the same basic movement from the floor, (lifting your torso and then lowering).

CRUNCH ON THE BALL

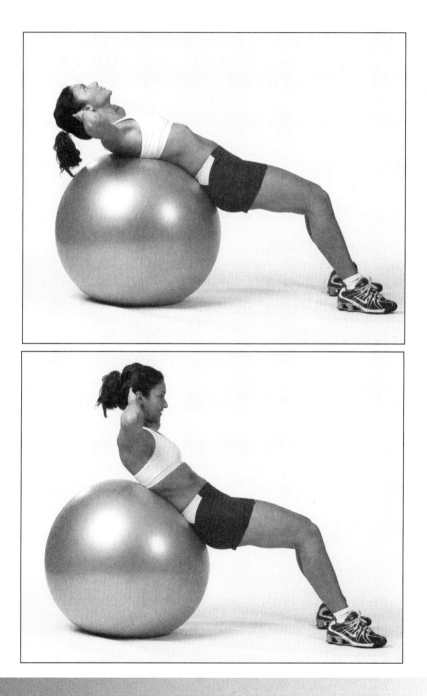

REVERSE CRUNCH WITH LEGS EXTENDED

Here's a great exercise for your overall core; if you are new to it, you may modify by keeping your legs bent.

TECHNIQUE AND FORM

1 Lie on the floor, grasping a fitness ball with your lower legs.

2 As you exhale, bring your legs up until they are perpendicular to the floor.

3 Slowly lower your legs until they are a few inches from the floor.

4 Hold for a count before repeating for desired number of repetitions.

TRAINER'S TIPS

To relieve pressure on your lower back, place your hands beneath your back.

If the exercise still strains your lower back, perform it with your knees bent instead of straight.

Keep your head on the mat for the duration of this exercise.

As you progress, when your legs reach the perpendicular position you can lift your torso and "catch" the ball with your hands, before returning it to the position between your legs and lowering.

REVERSE CRUNCH WITH LEGS EXTENDED

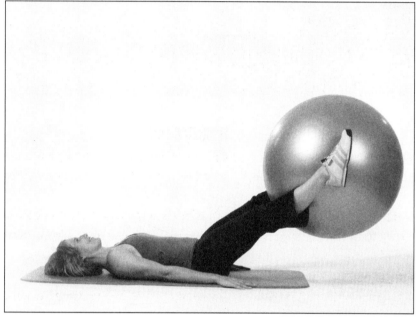

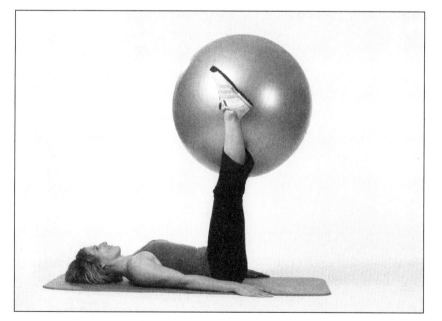

TWIST ON THE BALL

This is an exercise that maximizes recruitment of your obliques while also working the entire core. If you do not have a fitness ball, perform this exercise on a mat, keeping your shoulders elevated throughout the exercise as you twist from side to side.

TECHNIQUE AND FORM

1 Position yourself on the ball so that your lower back is supported. Your arms should be bent at the elbows and your head should be relaxed into the palms of your hands.

2 As you exhale, lift your chest and, leading with your right shoulder, twist over to your left knee.

3 Hold for a count until returning to the starting position.

4 Lift and twist, leading with your left shoulder, to your right knee.

5 Return to the start position.

6 Repeat for the desired number of repetitions, alternating the leading shoulder on each rep.

TRAINER'S TIPS

 Make sure that you are leading with your shoulder and not pulling on your neck. Your chest should be open.

 To increase the challenge of this exercise, lift your opposite leg off the ball as you perform the twist.

TWIST ON THE BALL

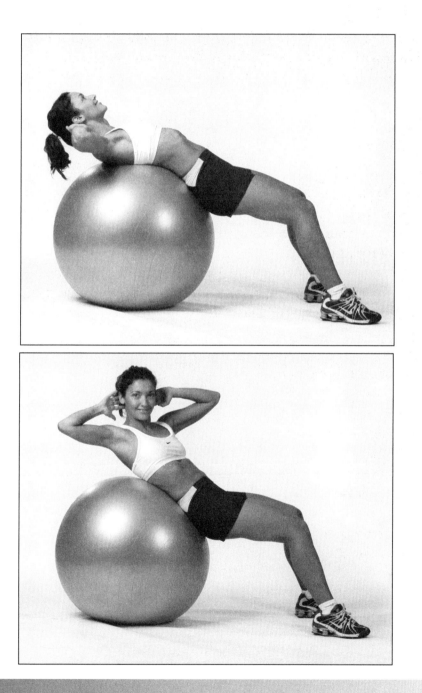

JACKKNIFE ON THE BALL

Here's an advanced exercise that requires upper body strength as well as a strong midsection.

TECHNIQUE AND FORM

1 Get into a push-up position, with your feet and lower legs resting on a fitness ball. Your hands should be on the floor, shoulder-width apart.

2 Pull your abs in as you bend your knees and bring your legs in to your chest. Your hips should lift to the ceiling. As you do this, exhale and curve your back to engage the abdominals.

3 Hold the top position for a count, before straightening back to the starting position.

4 Repeat for the desired number of repetitions.

TRAINER'S TIPS

✦ It is essential that you keep your abs pulled in and your glutes tight to keep your back flat (this avoids back strain.)

✦ To maximize muscle fiber recruitment, think about your abdominals as you pull the ball toward you.

✦ Release the contraction slowly, with control.

JACKKNIFE ON THE BALL

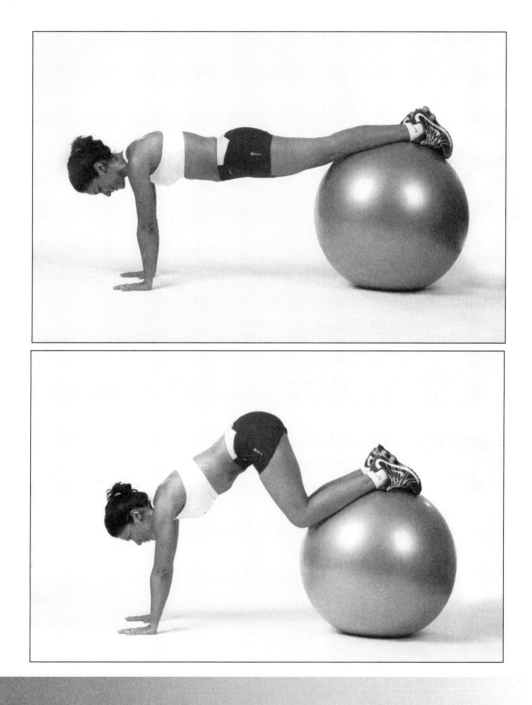

PLANK WITH ROTATION

A toughie, this exercise requires significant core (ab/back) strength. Work up to it.

TECHNIQUE AND FORM

1 Face the floor with your arms extended and shoulder-width apart, pull in your abdominals and squeeze your glutes to keep your back flat. Hold that plank position for a couple of seconds.

2 Lift your right arm off the floor and rotate your body so that you are balancing on your left arm and left foot.

3 Rotate back and return your right hand to the floor.

4 Exhale and lift your left arm off the floor and rotating your body so that you are balancing on your right side.

5 Repeat for desired number of repetitions.

TRAINER'S TIPS

  If the straight-arm plank is too difficult for you, you may perform this exercise with your forearms in contact with the floor.

  Think about using your abs and lower back muscles to stabilize your body as you lift. Also think about grounding your body with the opposite arm and leg.

PLANK WITH ROTATION

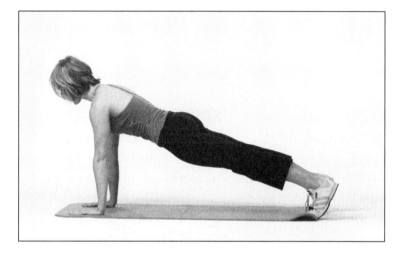

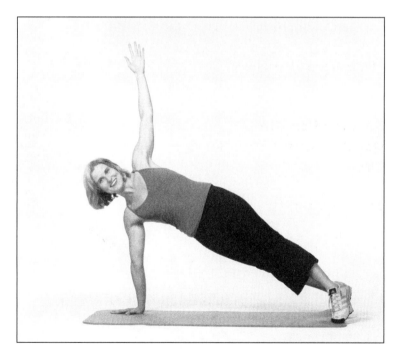

REVERSE CRUNCH

The reverse crunch targets the lower part of the abdominals.

TECHNIQUE AND FORM

1 Lie on a mat with your legs bent and raised from the floor.

2 Exhale and lift your hips slightly, bringing your knees in toward your chest. At the same time, lift your chest to meet your knees.

3 Hold the contraction for a second or two before releasing back to the start position.

4 Repeat for the desired number of repetitions.

TRAINER'S TIPS

Focus on pressing your belly button down into your spine at the same time as you lift your hips.

REVERSE CRUNCH

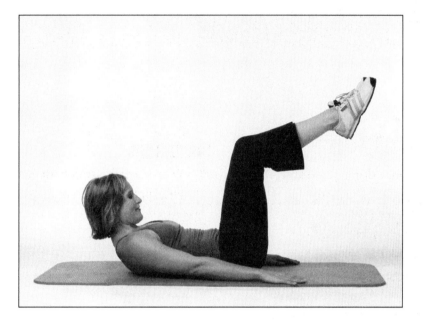

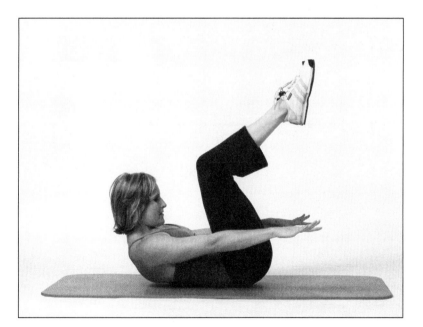

CRUNCH/PELVIC LIFT COMBINATION

This exercise targets both the outer and inner abdominals.

TECHNIQUE AND FORM

1 Lie on your back with your legs extended so that the soles of your feet face the ceiling. (Your legs should make a 90-degree angle with your body). Bend your arms behind your head.

2 As you exhale, slowly lift your torso, keeping your head in line with your spine.

3 At the same time, press your heels up to the ceiling by pressing your abs deep down through your spine.

4 Hold at the top position for a count or two before returning to a point where your shoulders don't quite touch the floor.

5 Repeat for the desired number of repetitions.

TRAINER'S TIPS

Make sure you keep your head back and that your neck is relaxed.

Try not to bring your shoulders down to the floor for the entire set. By keeping them slightly elevated you maintain tension and work the muscles throughout the range of motion.

For the pelvic lift segment of the exercise it is important that you mentally focus on the lower part of your abdominals and that you minimize action in the hips. The movement is very small—your buttocks should rise just an inch or two from the floor.

CRUNCH/PELVIC LIFT COMBINATION

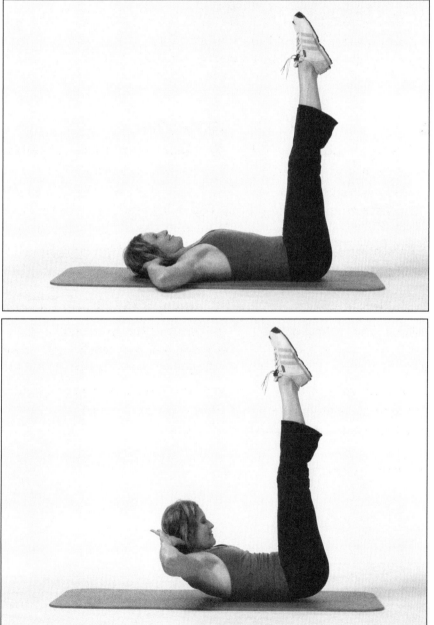

LOWER BACK EXTENSION

A great exercise to increase strength and support in your lower back; just be careful to not come up too high.

TECHNIQUE AND FORM

1 Lie on your stomach, with your legs extended and your head in line with your spine. Your arms should be straight down at your sides.

2 Exhale and slowly lift your torso and your legs simultaneously until you feel some pressure in your back.

3 Hold the top position for a couple of counts before returning to the starting position.

4 Repeat for the desired number of repetitions.

TRAINER'S TIPS

Be sure to lift only to the point of feeling some pressure in your lower back—if you feel any pain you are coming up too high and risking injury.

You can modify this exercise by lifting just the torso and keeping the legs in contact with the floor.

Another, more difficult variation is to perform this exercise with your arms extended over your head.

LOWER BACK EXTENSION

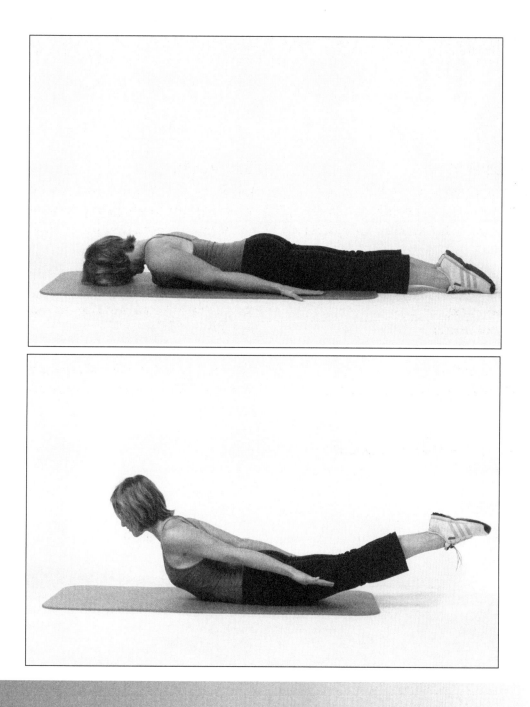

Part 3

The Workouts

Here they are. This part features three levels of Buns & Legs Workouts: Beginner, Intermediate, and Advanced. It also includes guidelines for cardiovascular workouts and suggestions to include upper body exercises on certain days.

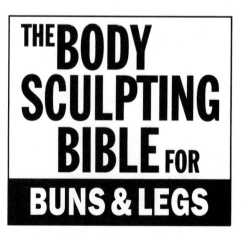

THE BODY SCULPTING BIBLE FOR BUNS & LEGS

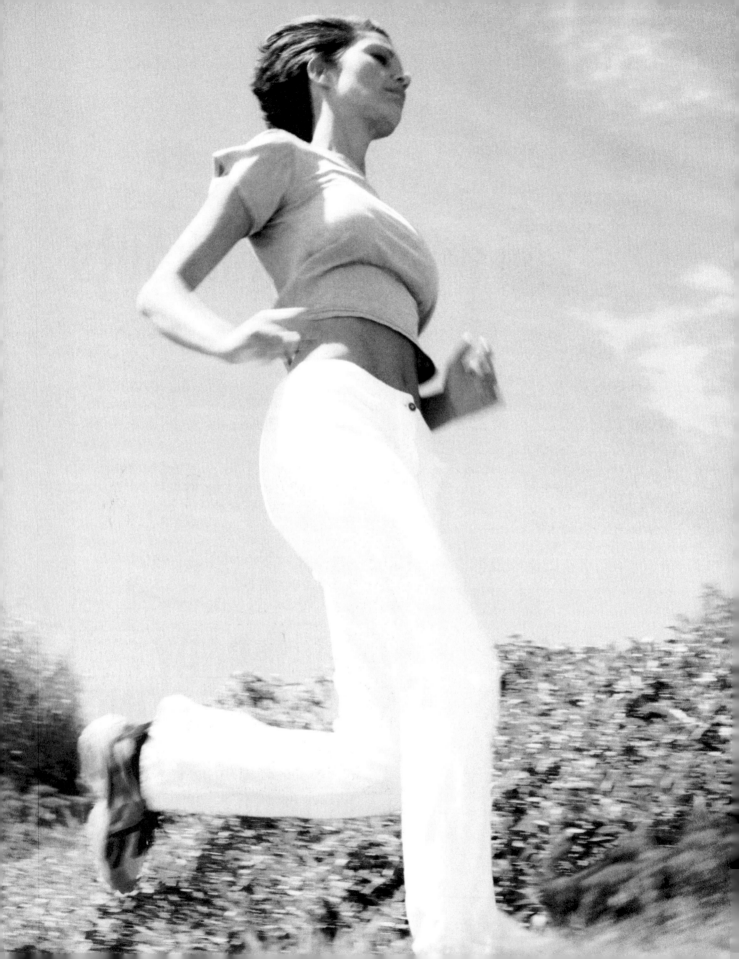

Chapter 8
Beginner Workout

The Beginner Workout involves performing exercises in pairs of modified compound supersets, and working opposing muscle groups in each pair. Every two weeks, the program changes to ensure your muscles remain challenged.

Choose this workout program if you have been working out with weights for less than three months, or if you are recovering from an injury. Check with your physician before beginning your exercise program. You will be working out three days a week, two of which focus on the lower body.

This workout's goals are to ease you into weight training safely and improve your muscle mass, definition, and overall body condition. This workout will also prepare you for the tougher ones that are yet to come.

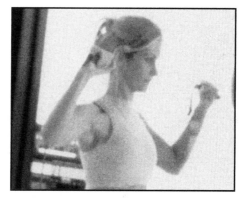

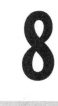

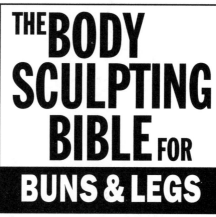

THE **BODY SCULPTING BIBLE** FOR **BUNS & LEGS**

WEEKS 1 & 2

DAY 1				MONDAY
EXERCISE	**PAGE NO.**	**REPS**	**SETS**	**REST**
MODIFIED COMPOUND SUPERSET # 1				
Glutes and Quads: Dumbbell Squat	48	12–15	2	60 seconds
Hamstrings: Lying Hamstring Curl on Machine	100	12–15	2	60 seconds
MODIFIED COMPOUND SUPERSET # 2				
Glutes and Quads: Leg Press on Machine	62	12–15	2	60 seconds
Hamstrings: Seated Leg Curl	106	12–15	2	60 seconds
MODIFIED COMPOUND SUPERSET # 3				
Outer Thigh: Side Lying Outer Thigh Leg Raise	84	12–15	2	60 seconds
Inner Thigh: Side Lying Leg Raise	70	12–15	2	60 seconds
MODIFIED COMPOUND SUPERSET # 4				
Calves: Calf Raise	112	12–15	2	60 seconds
Calves: Calf Press on Leg Press Machine	110	12–15	2	60 seconds
ABS WORKOUT				
Crunch on the Ball	122	15	2	30 seconds
Reverse Crunch with Legs Extended	124	15	2	30 seconds
Twist on the Ball	126	15	2	30 seconds
Crunch/Pelvic Lift Combination	134	15	2	30 seconds
Lower Back Extension	136	15	2	30 seconds

Cardio: Follow with 15 minutes of cardiovascular exercise such as elliptical, stationary bike, treadmill, or any other activity that will raise your heart rate to at least (220 – (Your Age)) x 0.75 +/– 10 beats.

WEEKS 1 & 2

DAY 2				WEDNESDAY
EXERCISE	**PAGE NO.**	**REPS**	**SETS**	**REST**
AB WORKOUT				
Crunch on the Ball	122	15	2	30 seconds
Reverse Crunch with Legs Extended	124	15	2	30 seconds
Twist on the Ball	126	15	2	30 seconds
Crunch/Pelvic Lift Combination	134	15	2	30 seconds
Lower Back Extension	136	15	2	30 seconds

Follow with an upper body routine, such as the one presented in the original *Body Sculpting Bible for Women* followed by 15 minutes of cardiovascular exercise such as elliptical, stationary bike, treadmill, or any other activity that will raise your heart rate to at least (220 – (Your Age)) x 0.75 +/– 10 beats. For your upper body training just follow the same repetition and rest schemes as the ones used for your lower body workouts.

DAY 3				FRIDAY
EXERCISE	**PAGE NO.**	**REPS**	**SETS**	**REST**
MODIFIED COMPOUND SUPERSET # 1				
Glutes and Quads: Wide Stance Squat	80	12–15	2	60 seconds
Hamstrings: Standing Hamstring Curl	104	12–15	2	60 seconds
MODIFIED COMPOUND SUPERSET # 2				
Glutes and Quads: Butt Blaster on Machine	66	12–15	2	60 seconds
Hamstrings: Deadlift	108	12–15	2	60 seconds
MODIFIED COMPOUND SUPERSET # 3				
Outer Thigh: Abductor on Machine	92	12–15	2	60 seconds
Inner Thigh: Adductor on Machine	76	12–15	2	60 seconds
MODIFIED COMPOUND SUPERSET # 4				
Calves: Seated Calf Raise	114	12–15	2	60 seconds
Calves: One-Legged Calf Press on Leg Press Machine	116	12–15	2	60 seconds
CARDIO AND ABS WORKOUT				
Crunch on the Ball	122	15	2	30 seconds
Reverse Crunch with Legs Extended	124	15	2	30 seconds
Twist on the Ball	126	15	2	30 seconds
Crunch/Pelvic Lift Combination	134	15	2	30 seconds
Lower Back Extension	136	15	2	30 seconds

Cardio: Follow with 15 minutes of cardiovascular exercise such as elliptical, stationary bike, treadmill, or any other activity that will raise your heart rate to at least (220 – (Your Age)) x 0.75 +/– 10 beats.

WEEKS 3 & 4

SPECIAL INSTRUCTIONS: Use pairs of modified compound supersets and decrease rest period to 45 seconds.

DAY 1				MONDAY
EXERCISE	**PAGE NO.**	**REPS**	**SETS**	**REST**
MODIFIED COMPOUND SUPERSET # 1				
Glutes and Quads: Dumbbell Squat	48	12–15	2	45 seconds
Hamstrings: Lying Hamstring Curl on Machine	100	12–15	2	45 seconds
MODIFIED COMPOUND SUPERSET # 2				
Glutes and Quads: Leg Press on Machine	62	12–15	2	45 seconds
Hamstrings: Seated Leg Curl	106	12–15	2	45 seconds
MODIFIED COMPOUND SUPERSET # 3				
Outer Thigh: Side Lying Outer Thigh Leg Raise	84	12–15	2	45 seconds
Inner Thigh: Side Lying Leg Raise	70	12–15	2	45 seconds
MODIFIED COMPOUND SUPERSET # 4				
Calves: Calf Raise	112	12–15	2	45 seconds
Calves: Calf Press on Leg Press Machine	110	12–15	2	45 seconds
ABS WORKOUT				
Crunch on the Ball	122	15	2	30 seconds
Reverse Crunch with Legs Extended	124	15	2	30 seconds
Twist on the Ball	126	15	2	30 seconds
Crunch/Pelvic Lift Combination	134	15	2	30 seconds
Lower Back Extension	136	15	2	30 seconds
Cardio: Follow with 15 minutes of cardiovascular exercise such as elliptical, stationary bike, treadmill, or any other activity that will raise your heart rate to at least (220 – (Your Age)) x 0.75 +/– 10 beats.				

WEEKS 3 & 4

DAY 2				WEDNESDAY
EXERCISE	**PAGE NO.**	**REPS**	**SETS**	**REST**
AB WORKOUT				
Crunch on the Ball	122	15	2	30 seconds
Reverse Crunch with Legs Extended	124	15	2	30 seconds
Twist on the Ball	126	15	2	30 seconds
Crunch/Pelvic Lift Combination	134	15	2	30 seconds
Lower Back Extension	136	15	2	30 seconds

Follow with an upper body routine, such as the one presented in the original *Body Sculpting Bible for Women* followed by 15 minutes of cardiovascular exercise such as elliptical, stationary bike, treadmill, or any other activity that will raise your heart rate to at least (220 – (Your Age)) x 0.75 +/– 10 beats. For your upper body training just follow the same repetition and rest schemes as the ones used for your lower body workouts.

DAY 3				FRIDAY
EXERCISE	**PAGE NO.**	**REPS**	**SETS**	**REST**
MODIFIED COMPOUND SUPERSET # 1				
Glutes and Quads: Wide Stance Squat	80	12–15	2	45 seconds
Hamstrings: Standing Hamstring Curl	104	12–15	2	45 seconds
MODIFIED COMPOUND SUPERSET # 2				
Glutes and Quads: Butt Blaster on Machine	66	12–15	2	45 seconds
Hamstrings: Deadlift	108	12–15	2	45 seconds
MODIFIED COMPOUND SUPERSET # 3				
Outer Thigh: Abductor on Machine	92	12–15	2	45 seconds
Inner Thigh: Adductor on Machine	76	12–15	2	45 seconds
MODIFIED COMPOUND SUPERSET # 4				
Calves: Seated Calf Raise	114	12–15	2	45 seconds
Calves: One-Legged Calf Press on Leg Press Machine	116	12–15	2	45 seconds
ABS WORKOUT				
Crunch on the Ball	122	15	2	30 seconds
Reverse Crunch with Legs Extended	124	15	2	30 seconds
Twist on the Ball	126	15	2	30 seconds
Crunch/Pelvic Lift Combination	134	15	2	30 seconds
Lower Back Extension	136	15	2	30 seconds

Cardio: Follow with 15 minutes of cardiovascular exercise such as elliptical, stationary bike, treadmill, or any other activity that will raise your heart rate to at least (220 – (Your Age)) x 0.75 +/– 10 beats.

WEEKS 5 & 6

SPECIAL INSTRUCTIONS: Use pairs of modified compound supersets. Increase weight to allow for 10 to 12 rep maximum per set.

DAY 1				MONDAY
EXERCISE	**PAGE NO.**	**REPS**	**SETS**	**REST**
MODIFIED COMPOUND SUPERSET # 1				
Glutes and Quads: Dumbbell Squat	48	10–12	2	45 seconds
Hamstrings: Lying Hamstring Curl on Machine	100	10–12	2	45 seconds
MODIFIED COMPOUND SUPERSET # 2				
Glutes and Quads: Leg Press on Machine	62	10–12	2	45 seconds
Hamstrings: Seated Leg Curl	106	10–12	2	45 seconds
MODIFIED COMPOUND SUPERSET # 3				
Outer Thigh: Side Lying Outer Thigh Leg Raise	84	10–12	2	45 seconds
Inner Thigh: Side Lying Leg Raise	70	10–12	2	45 seconds
MODIFIED COMPOUND SUPERSET # 4				
Calves: Calf Raise	112	10–12	2	45 seconds
Calves: Calf Press on Leg Press Machine	110	10–12	2	45 seconds
ABS WORKOUT				
Crunch on the Ball	122	15	2	30 seconds
Reverse Crunch with Legs Extended	124	15	2	30 seconds
Twist on the Ball	126	15	2	30 seconds
Crunch/Pelvic Lift Combination	134	15	2	30 seconds
Lower Back Extension	136	15	2	30 seconds

Cardio: Follow with 15 minutes of cardiovascular exercise such as elliptical, stationary bike, treadmill, or any other activity that will raise your heart rate to at least (220 – (Your Age)) x 0.75 +/– 10 beats.

WEEKS 5 & 6

DAY 2				WEDNESDAY
EXERCISE	**PAGE NO.**	**REPS**	**SETS**	**REST**
AB WORKOUT				
Crunch on the Ball	122	15	2	30 seconds
Reverse Crunch with Legs Extended	124	15	2	30 seconds
Twist on the Ball	126	15	2	30 seconds
Crunch/Pelvic Lift Combination	134	15	2	30 seconds
Lower Back Extension	136	15	2	30 seconds

Follow with an upper body routine, such as the one presented in the original *Body Sculpting Bible for Women* followed by 15 minutes of cardiovascular exercise such as elliptical, stationary bike, treadmill, or any other activity that will raise your heart rate to at least (220 – (Your Age)) x 0.75 +/– 10 beats. For your upper body training just follow the same repetition and rest schemes as the ones used for your lower body workouts.

DAY 3				FRIDAY
EXERCISE	**PAGE NO.**	**REPS**	**SETS**	**REST**
MODIFIED COMPOUND SUPERSET # 1				
Glutes and Quads: Wide Stance Squat	80	10–12	2	45 seconds
Hamstrings: Standing Hamstring Curl	104	10–12	2	45 seconds
MODIFIED COMPOUND SUPERSET # 2				
Glutes and Quads: Butt Blaster on Machine	66	10–12	2	45 seconds
Hamstrings: Deadlift	108	10–12	2	45 seconds
MODIFIED COMPOUND SUPERSET # 3				
Outer Thigh: Abductor on Machine	92	10–12	2	45 seconds
Inner Thigh: Adductor on Machine	76	10–12	2	45 seconds
MODIFIED COMPOUND SUPERSET # 4				
Calves: Seated Calf Raise	114	10–12	2	45 seconds
Calves: One-Legged Calf Press on Leg Press Machine	116	10–12	2	45 seconds
ABS WORKOUT				
Crunch on the Ball	122	15	2	30 seconds
Reverse Crunch with Legs Extended	124	15	2	30 seconds
Twist on the Ball	126	15	2	30 seconds
Crunch/Pelvic Lift Combination	134	15	2	30 seconds
Lower Back Extension	136	15	2	30 seconds

Cardio: Follow with 15 minutes of cardiovascular exercise such as elliptical, stationary bike, treadmill, or any other activity that will raise your heart rate to at least (220 – (Your Age)) x 0.75 +/– 10 beats.

WEEKS 7 & 8

SPECIAL INSTRUCTIONS: Use pairs of supersets. Remove rest in between exercises in each set. Increase to three sets per exercise.

DAY 1				MONDAY
EXERCISE	**PAGE NO.**	**REPS**	**SETS**	**REST**
MODIFIED COMPOUND SUPERSET # 1				
Glutes and Quads: Dumbbell Squat	48	10–12	3	0 seconds
Hamstrings: Lying Hamstring Curl on Machine	100	10–12	3	45 seconds
MODIFIED COMPOUND SUPERSET # 2				
Glutes and Quads: Leg Press on Machine	62	10–12	3	0 seconds
Hamstrings: Seated Leg Curl	106	10–12	3	45 seconds
MODIFIED COMPOUND SUPERSET # 3				
Outer Thigh: Side Lying Outer Thigh Leg Raise	84	10–12	3	0 seconds
Inner Thigh: Side Lying Leg Raise	70	10–12	3	45 seconds
MODIFIED COMPOUND SUPERSET # 4				
Calves: Calf Raise	112	10–12	3	0 seconds
Calves: Calf Press on Leg Press Machine	110	10–12	3	45 seconds
ABS WORKOUT				
Crunch on the Ball	122	15	3	30 seconds
Reverse Crunch with Legs Extended	124	15	3	30 seconds
Twist on the Ball	126	15	3	30 seconds
Crunch/Pelvic Lift Combination	134	15	3	30 seconds
Lower Back Extension	136	15	3	30 seconds

Cardio: Follow with 15 minutes of cardiovascular exercise such as elliptical, stationary bike, treadmill, or any other activity that will raise your heart rate to at least (220 – (Your Age)) x 0.75 +/– 10 beats.

WEEKS 7 & 8

DAY 2				WEDNESDAY
EXERCISE	**PAGE NO.**	**REPS**	**SETS**	**REST**
AB WORKOUT				
Crunch on the Ball	122	15	3	30 seconds
Reverse Crunch with Legs Extended	124	15	3	30 seconds
Twist on the Ball	126	15	3	30 seconds
Crunch/Pelvic Lift Combination	134	15	3	30 seconds
Lower Back Extension	136	15	3	30 seconds

Follow with an upper body routine, such as the one presented in the original *Body Sculpting Bible for Women* followed by 15 minutes of cardiovascular exercise such as elliptical, stationary bike, treadmill, or any other activity that will raise your heart rate to at least (220 – (Your Age)) x 0.75 +/– 10 beats. For your upper body training, just follow the same repetition and rest schemes as the ones used for your lower body workouts.

DAY 3				FRIDAY
EXERCISE	**PAGE NO.**	**REPS**	**SETS**	**REST**
MODIFIED COMPOUND SUPERSET # 1				
Glutes and Quads: Wide Stance Squat	80	10–12	3	0 seconds
Hamstrings: Standing Hamstring Curl	104	10–12	3	45 seconds
MODIFIED COMPOUND SUPERSET # 2				
Glutes and Quads: Butt Blaster on Machine	66	10–12	3	0 seconds
Hamstrings: Deadlift	108	10–12	3	45 seconds
MODIFIED COMPOUND SUPERSET # 3				
Outer Thigh: Abductor on Machine	92	10–12	3	0 seconds
Inner Thigh: Adductor on Machine	76	10–12	3	45 seconds
MODIFIED COMPOUND SUPERSET # 4				
Calves: Seated Calf Raise	114	10–12	3	0 seconds
Calves: One-Legged Calf Press on Leg Press Machine	116	10–12	3	45 seconds
ABS WORKOUT				
Crunch on the Ball	122	15	3	30 seconds
Reverse Crunch with Legs Extended	124	15	3	30 seconds
Twist on the Ball	126	15	3	30 seconds
Crunch/Pelvic Lift Combination	134	15	3	30 seconds
Lower Back Extension	136	15	3	30 seconds

Cardio: Follow with 15 minutes of cardiovascular exercise such as elliptical, stationary bike, treadmill, or any other activity that will raise your heart rate to at least (220 – (Your Age)) x 0.75 +/– 10 beats.

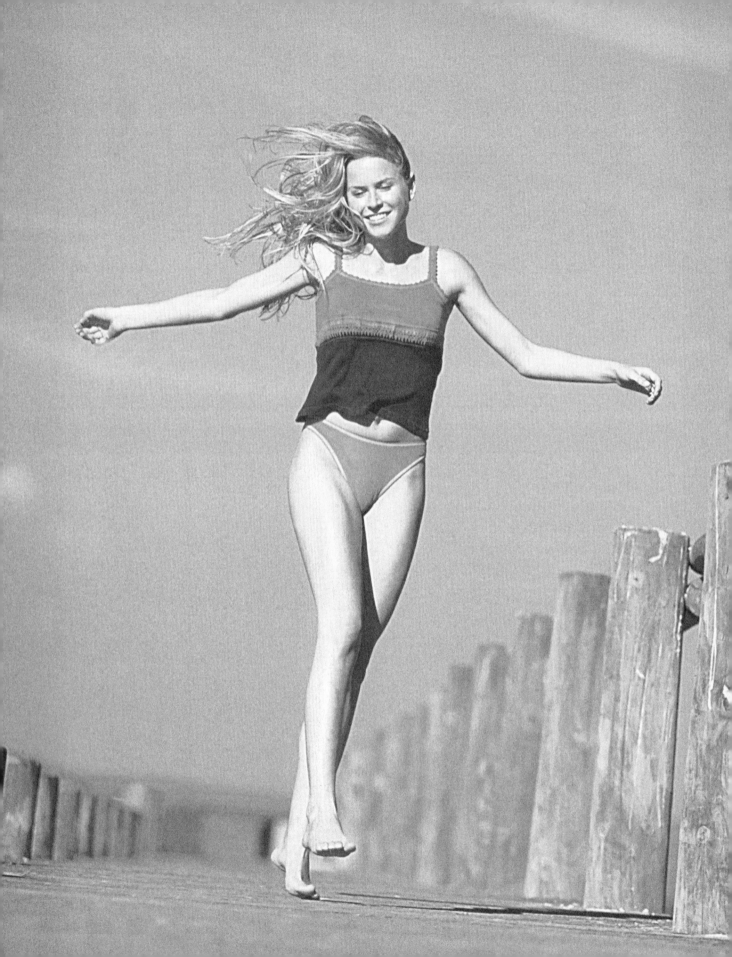

Chapter 9
Intermediate Workout

Choose the Intermediate Workout if you have been training for three months to one year. The goal of this program is to increase muscle definition with a moderate increase in muscle mass.

The Intermediate Workout program includes four workouts each week, two of which focus on the lower body.

The goals for this workout are to increase your muscle definition with a moderate increase in muscle mass.

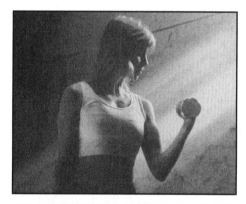

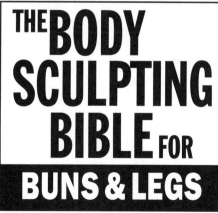

THE BODY SCULPTING BIBLE FOR BUNS & LEGS

9

WEEKS 1 & 2

SPECIAL INSTRUCTIONS: Perform 12 to 15 repetitions of each exercise and two sets. Note that the pace of the workout is fast as well, in order to emphasize definition.

DAY 1				MONDAY
EXERCISE	**PAGE NO.**	**REPS**	**SETS**	**REST**
MODIFIED COMPOUND SUPERSET # 1				
Glutes and Quads: Dumbbell Squat	48	12–15	2	30 seconds
Glutes and Quads: Multi–Directional Lunges	56	12–15	2	30 seconds
Glutes and Quads: Leg Press on Machine	62	12–15	2	30 seconds
Glutes and Quads: One-Legged Butt Press with Ball	60	12–15	2	60 seconds
MODIFIED COMPOUND SUPERSET # 2				
Outer Thighs: Cable Leg Raise for Outer Thigh	78	12–15	2	30 seconds
Outer Thighs: Squat with Abduction	90	12–15	2	30 seconds
Inner Thighs: Wide Stance Squat	80	12–15	2	30 seconds
Inner Thighs: Ball Extension	82	12–15	2	60 seconds
AB WORKOUT				
Crunch on the Ball	122	20	3	30 seconds
Reverse Crunch with Legs Extended	124	20	3	30 seconds
Twist on the Ball	126	20	3	30 seconds
Crunch/Pelvic Lift Combination	134	20	3	30 seconds
Reverse Crunch	132	20	3	30 seconds
Lower Back Extension	136	20	3	30 seconds

Cardio: Follow with 20 minutes of cardiovascular exercise such as elliptical, stationary bike, treadmill, or any other activity that will raise your heart rate to at least (220 – (Your Age)) x 0.75 +/– 10 beats.

DAYS 2 AND 4	WEDNESDAY AND SATURDAY

On Wednesdays and Saturdays you can perform an upper body workout, such as the one presented in *The Body Sculpting Bible for Women*, followed by 20 minutes of cardiovascular exercise such as elliptical, stationary bike, treadmill, or any other activity that will raise your heart rate to at least (220 – (Your Age)) x 0.75 +/– 10 beats. For your upper body training, just follow the same repetition and rest schemes as the ones used for your lower body workouts.

WEEKS 1 & 2

DAY 3				FRIDAY
EXERCISE	**PAGE NO.**	**REPS**	**SETS**	**REST**
MODIFIED COMPOUND SUPERSET # 1				
Glutes and Quads: One-Legged Squat	52	12–15	2	30 seconds
Glutes and Quads: Leg Extension Machine	64	12–15	2	30 seconds
Glutes and Quads: Ball Lunge	58	12–15	2	30 seconds
Glutes and Quads: Butt Blaster on Machine	66	12–15	2	60 seconds
MODIFIED COMPOUND SUPERSET #2				
Hamstrings: Hamstring Curl on the Ball	102	12–15	2	30 seconds
Hamstrings: Lying Hamstring Curl on Machine	100	12–15	2	30 seconds
Calves: Multi-Directional Calf Raises	118	12–15	2	30 seconds
Calves: Calf Press on Leg Press Machine	110	12–15	2	60 seconds
AB WORKOUT				
Crunch on the Ball	122	20	3	30 seconds
Reverse Crunch with Legs Extended	124	20	3	30 seconds
Twist on the Ball	126	20	3	30 seconds
Crunch/Pelvic Lift Combination	134	20	3	30 seconds
Reverse Crunch	132	20	3	30 seconds
Lower Back Extension	136	20	3	30 seconds

Cardio: Follow with 20 minutes of cardiovascular exercise such as elliptical, stationary bike, treadmill, or any other activity that will raise your heart rate to at least (220 – (Your Age)) x 0.75 +/– 10 beats.

WEEKS 3 & 4

SPECIAL INSTRUCTIONS: Perform 10 to 12 repetitions of each exercise and three sets. Eliminate the rest in between some of the exercises as prescribed below.

DAY 1				MONDAY
EXERCISE	**PAGE NO.**	**REPS**	**SETS**	**REST**
SUPERSET # 1				
Glutes and Quads: Dumbbell Squat	48	10–12	3	0 seconds
Glutes and Quads: Multi–Directional Lunges	50	10–12	3	30 seconds
Glutes and Quads: Leg Press on Machine	62	10–12	3	0 seconds
Glutes and Quads: One-Legged Butt Press with Ball	60	10–12	3	60 seconds
SUPERSET # 2				
Outer Thighs: Cable Leg Raise for Outer Thigh	86	10–12	3	0 seconds
Outer Thighs: Squat with Abduction	90	10–12	3	30 seconds
Inner Thighs: Wide Stance Squat	80	10–12	3	0 seconds
Inner Thighs: Ball Extension	82	10–12	3	60 seconds
AB WORKOUT				
Crunch on the Ball	122	20	3	30 seconds
Reverse Crunch with Legs Extended	124	20	3	30 seconds
Twist on the Ball	126	20	3	30 seconds
Crunch/Pelvic Lift Combination	134	20	3	30 seconds
Reverse Crunch	132	20	3	30 seconds
Lower Back Extension	136	20	3	30 seconds

Cardio: Follow with 30 minutes of cardiovascular exercise such as elliptical, stationary bike, treadmill, or any other activity that will raise your heart rate to at least (220 – (Your Age)) x 0.75 +/– 10 beats.

DAYS 2 AND 4	WEDNESDAY AND SATURDAY

On Wednesdays and Saturdays you can perform an upper body workout, such as the one presented in *The Body Sculpting Bible for Women*, followed by 20 minutes of cardiovascular exercise such as elliptical, stationary bike, treadmill, or any other activity that will raise your heart rate to at least (220 – (Your Age)) x 0.75 +/– 10 beats. For your upper body training, just follow the same repetition and rest schemes as the ones used for your lower body workouts.

WEEKS 3 & 4

DAY 3				FRIDAY
EXERCISE	**PAGE NO.**	**REPS**	**SETS**	**REST**
SUPERSET # 1				
Glutes and Quads: One-Legged Squat	52	10–12	3	0 seconds
Glutes and Quads: Leg Extension Machine	64	10–12	3	30 seconds
Glutes and Quads: Ball Lunge	58	10–12	3	0 seconds
Glutes and Quads: Butt Blaster on Machine	66	10–12	3	60 seconds
SUPERSET # 2				
Hamstrings: Hamstring Curl on the Ball	102	10–12	3	0 seconds
Hamstrings: Lying Hamstring Curl on Machine	100	10–12	3	30 seconds
Calves: Multi–Directional Calf Raises	118	10–12	3	0 seconds
Calves: Calf Press on Leg Press Machine	110	10–12	3	60 seconds
AB WORKOUT				
Crunch on the Ball	122	20	3	30 seconds
Reverse Crunch with Legs Extended	124	20	3	30 seconds
Twist on the Ball	126	20	3	30 seconds
Crunch/Pelvic Lift Combination	134	20	3	30 seconds
Reverse Crunch	132	20	3	30 seconds
Lower Back Extension	136	20	3	30 seconds

Cardio: Follow with 30 minutes of cardiovascular exercise such as elliptical, stationary bike, treadmill, or any other activity that will raise your heart rate to at least (220 – (Your Age)) x 0.75 +/– 10 beats.

WEEKS 5 & 6

SPECIAL INSTRUCTIONS: Perform 8 to 10 repetitions of each exercise. Perform the exercises as Giant Sets, removing the rest period between exercises.

DAY 1				MONDAY
EXERCISE	**PAGE NO.**	**REPS**	**SETS**	**REST**
GIANT SET # 1				
Glutes and Quads: Dumbbell Squat	48	8–10	3	0 seconds
Glutes and Quads: Multi–Directional Lunges	50	8–10	3	0 seconds
Glutes and Quads: Leg Press on Machine	62	8–10	3	0 seconds
Glutes and Quads: One-Legged Butt Press with Ball	60	8–10	3	60 seconds
GIANT SET # 2				
Outer Thighs: Cable Leg Raise for Outer Thigh	86	8–10	3	0 seconds
Outer Thighs: Squat with Abduction	90	8–10	3	0 seconds
Inner Thighs: Wide Stance Squat	80	8–10	3	0 seconds
Inner Thighs: Ball Extension	82	8–10	3	60 seconds
AB WORKOUT				
Crunch on the Ball	122	20	3	30 seconds
Reverse Crunch with Legs Extended	124	20	3	30 seconds
Twist on the Ball	126	20	3	30 seconds
Crunch/Pelvic Lift Combination	134	20	3	30 seconds
Reverse Crunch	132	20	3	30 seconds
Lower Back Extension	136	20	3	30 seconds

Cardio: Follow with 40 minutes of cardiovascular exercise such as elliptical, stationary bike, treadmill, or any other activity that will raise your heart rate to at least (220 – (Your Age)) x 0.75 +/– 10 beats.

DAYS 2 AND 4	WEDNESDAY AND SATURDAY

On Wednesdays and Saturdays you can perform an upper body workout, such as the one presented in in *The Body Sculpting Bible for Women* followed by 40 minutes of cardiovascular exercise such as elliptical, stationary bike, treadmill, or any other activity that will raise your heart rate to at least (220 – (Your Age)) x 0.75 +/– 10 beats. For your upper body training, just follow the same repetition and rest schemes as the ones used for your lower body workouts.

WEEKS 5 & 6

DAY 3				FRIDAY
EXERCISE	**PAGE NO.**	**REPS**	**SETS**	**REST**
GIANT SET # 1				
Glutes and Quads: One-Legged Squat	52	8–10	3	0 seconds
Glutes and Quads: Leg Extension Machine	64	8–10	3	0 seconds
Glutes and Quads: Ball Lunge	58	8–10	3	0 seconds
Glutes and Quads: Butt Blaster on Machine	66	8–10	3	60 seconds
GIANT SET # 2				
Hamstrings: Hamstring Curl on the Ball	102	8–10	3	0 seconds
Hamstrings: Lying Hamstring Curl on Machine	100	8–10	3	0 seconds
Calves: Multi-Directional Calf Raises	118	8–10	3	0 seconds
Calves: Calf Press on Leg Press Machine	110	8–10	3	60 seconds
AB WORKOUT				
Crunch on the Ball	122	20	3	30 seconds
Reverse Crunch with Legs Extended	124	20	3	30 seconds
Twist on the Ball	126	20	3	30 seconds
Crunch/Pelvic Lift Combination	134	20	3	30 seconds
Reverse Crunch	132	20	3	30 seconds
Lower Back Extension	136	20	3	30 seconds

Cardio: Follow with 40 minutes of cardiovascular exercise such as elliptical, stationary bike, treadmill, or any other activity that will raise your heart rate to at least (220 – (Your Age)) x 0.75 +/– 10 beats.

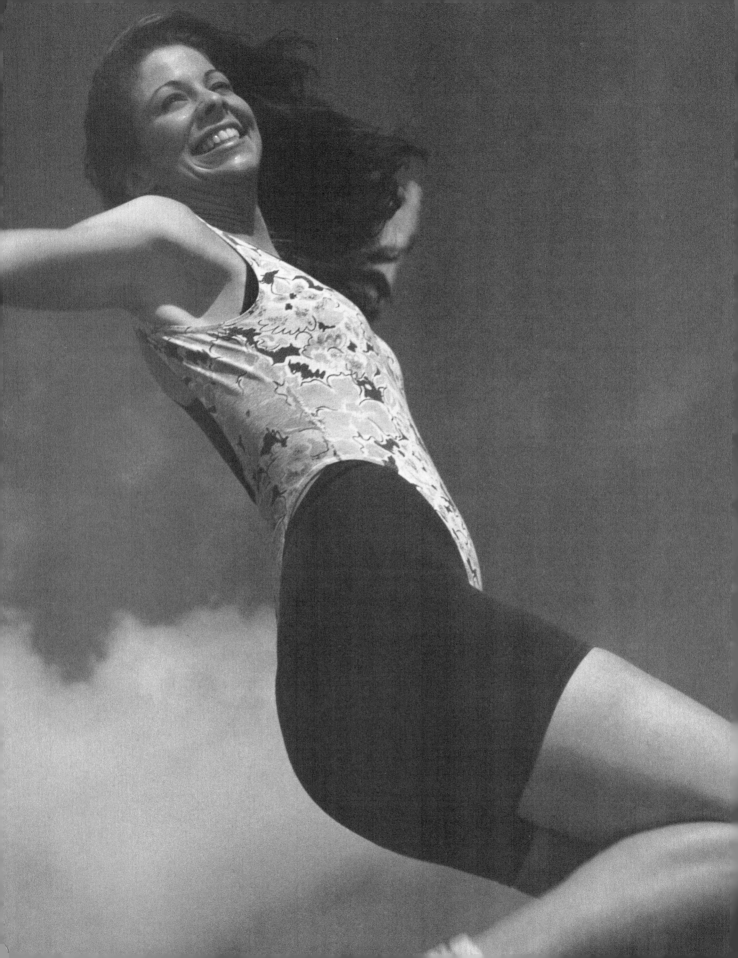

Chapter 10
Advanced Workout

The Advanced Workout is a challenging intense body-shaper for those of you with more than one year's training. It consists of 6 workouts each week, 3 of which target the lower body.

The goals for this workout are to increase your muscle definition with a slight increase in muscle mass. This workout will get your legs in the best shape possible when used in conjunction with the nutrition program offered in Chapter 2. Please do not jump into this routine unless you have at least a year of training under your belt.

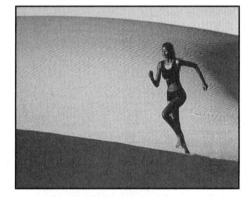

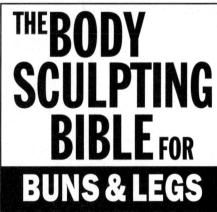

THE **BODY SCULPTING BIBLE** FOR

BUNS & LEGS

10

WEEKS 1 & 2

SPECIAL INSTRUCTIONS: Perform 12 to 15 repetitions of each exercise and two or three sets. Note that the pace of the workout is a bit slower and that the repetition ranges are also lower in order to emphasize muscle mass. In addition, the exercises selected recruit the most muscle fibers in order to get the most muscle mass gains in the shortest amount of time.

DAY 1				MONDAY
EXERCISE	**PAGE NO.**	**REPS**	**SETS**	**REST**
MODIFIED COMPOUND SUPERSET # 1				
Glutes and Quads: Dumbbell Squat	48	12–15	3	60 seconds
Hamstrings: Hamstring Curl on the Ball	102	12–15	3	60 seconds
Glutes and Quads: Multi-Directional Lunges	50	12–15	3	60 seconds
Hamstrings: Deadlift	108	12–15	3	60 seconds
MODIFIED COMPOUND SUPERSET # 2				
Outer Thighs: Ball Abduction	94	12–15	3	60 seconds
Inner Thighs: Lateral Lunge onto BOSU or Step	74	12–15	3	60 seconds
Outer Thighs: Abductor on Machine	92	12–15	3	60 seconds
Inner Thighs: Adductor on Machine	76	12–15	3	60 seconds
AB WORKOUT				
Crunch on the Ball	122	20	2	15 seconds
Reverse Crunch with Legs Extended	124	20	2	15 seconds
Twist on the Ball	126	20	2	15 seconds
Jackknife on the Ball	128	20	2	15 seconds
Reverse Crunch	132	20	2	15 seconds
Plank with Rotation	130	20	2	15 seconds
Lower Back Extension	136	20	2	15 seconds

Cardio: Follow with 20 minutes of cardiovascular exercise such as elliptical, stationary bike, treadmill, or any other activity that will raise your heart rate to at least (220 – (Your Age)) x 0.75 +/– 10 beats.

DAYS 2, 4, AND 6	TUESDAY, THURSDAY, AND SATURDAY

On Tuesdays, Thursdays, and Saturdays you can perform an upper body workout, such as the one presented in *The Body Sculpting Bible for Women* followed by 20 minutes of cardiovascular exercise such as elliptical, stationary bike, treadmill, or any other activity that will raise your heart rate to at least (220 – (Your Age)) x 0.75 +/– 10 beats. For your upper body training, just follow the same repetition and rest schemes as the ones used for your lower body workouts.

DAY 3 — WEDNESDAY

EXERCISE	PAGE NO.	REPS	SETS	REST
MODIFIED COMPOUND SUPERSET # 1				
Glutes and Quads: One-Legged Squat with Ball	56	12–15	3	60 seconds
Hamstrings: Lying Hamstring Curl on Machine	100	12–15	3	60 seconds
Glutes and Quads: Ball Lunge	58	12–15	3	60 seconds
Hamstrings: Curl On All Fours	98	12–15	3	60 seconds
MODIFIED COMPOUND SUPERSET # 2				
Outer Thighs: Cable Leg Raise for Outer Thigh	86	12–15	3	60 seconds
Inner Thighs: Cable Leg Raise	78	12–15	3	60 seconds
Calves: Multi-Directional Calf Raises	118	12–15	3	60 seconds
Calves: Calf Press on Leg Press Machine	110	12–15	3	60 seconds
AB WORKOUT				
Crunch on the Ball	122	20	2	15 seconds
Reverse Crunch with Legs Extended	124	20	2	15 seconds
Twist on the Ball	126	20	2	15 seconds
Jackknife on the Ball	128	20	2	15 seconds
Reverse Crunch	132	20	2	15 seconds
Plank with Rotation	130	20	2	15 seconds
Lower Back Extension	136	20	2	15 seconds

Cardio: Follow with 20 minutes of cardiovascular exercise such as elliptical, stationary bike, treadmill, or any other activity that will raise your heart rate to at least (220 – (Your Age)) x 0.75 +/– 10 beats.

DAY 5 — FRIDAY

EXERCISE	PAGE NO.	REPS	SETS	REST
MODIFIED COMPOUND SUPERSET # 1				
Glutes and Quads: Leg Press on Machine	62	12–15	3	60 seconds
Hamstrings: Hamstring Curl on the Ball	102	12–15	3	60 seconds
Glutes and Quads: One-Legged Butt Press with Ball	60	12–15	3	60 seconds
Hamstrings: Curl On All Fours	98	12–15	3	60 seconds
MODIFIED COMPOUND SUPERSET # 2				
Outer Thighs: Squat with Abduction	90	12–15	3	60 seconds
Inner Thighs: Lateral Lunge	72	12–15	3	60 seconds
Outer Thighs: Side Leg Kick	88	12–15	3	60 seconds
Inner Thighs: Wide Stance Squat	80	12–15	3	60 seconds
AB WORKOUT				
Crunch on the Ball	122	20	2	15 seconds
Reverse Crunch with Legs Extended	124	20	2	15 seconds
Twist on the Ball	126	20	2	15 seconds
Jackknife on the Ball	128	20	2	15 seconds
Reverse Crunch	132	20	2	15 seconds
Plank with Rotation	130	20	2	15 seconds
Lower Back Extension	136	20	2	15 seconds

Cardio: Follow with 20 minutes of cardiovascular exercise such as elliptical, stationary bike, treadmill, or any other activity that will raise your heart rate to at least (220 – (Your Age)) x 0.75 +/– 10 beats.

WEEKS 3 & 4

SPECIAL INSTRUCTIONS: Perform 10 to 12 repetitions of each exercise as noted below. Eliminate the rest in between some of the exercises as prescribed below.

DAY 1				MONDAY
EXERCISE	**PAGE NO.**	**REPS**	**SETS**	**REST**
SUPERSET # 1				
Glutes and Quads: Dumbbell Squat	48	10–12	4	0 seconds
Hamstrings: Hamstring Curl on the Ball	102	10–12	4	60 seconds
Glutes and Quads: Multi–Directional Lunges	50	10–12	4	0 seconds
Hamstrings: Deadlift	108	10–12	4	60 seconds
SUPERSET # 2				
Outer Thighs: Ball Abduction	94	10–12	4	0 seconds
Inner Thighs: Lateral Lunge onto BOSU or Step	74	10–12	4	60 seconds
Outer Thighs: Abductor on Machine	92	10–12	4	0 seconds
Inner Thighs: Adductor on Machine	76	10–12	4	60 seconds
AB WORKOUT				
Crunch on the Ball	122	20	2	15 seconds
Reverse Crunch with Legs Extended	124	20	2	15 seconds
Twist on the Ball	126	20	2	15 seconds
Jackknife on the Ball	128	20	2	15 seconds
Reverse Crunch	132	20	2	15 seconds
Plank with Rotation	130	20	2	15 seconds
Lower Back Extension	136	20	2	15 seconds

Cardio: Follow with 30 minutes of cardiovascular exercise such as elliptical, stationary bike, treadmill, or any other activity that will raise your heart rate to at least (220 – (Your Age)) x 0.75 +/– 10 beats.

DAYS 2, 4, AND 6	TUESDAY, THURSDAY, AND SATURDAY

On Tuesdays, Thursdays, and Saturdays you can perform an upper body workout, such as the one presented in in *The Body Sculpting Bible for Women* followed by 30 minutes of cardiovascular exercise such as elliptical, stationary bike, treadmill, or any other activity that will raise your heart rate to at least (220 – (Your Age)) x 0.75 +/– 10 beats. For your upper body training, just follow the same repetition and rest schemes as the ones used for your lower-body workouts.

DAY 3 — WEDNESDAY

EXERCISE	PAGE NO.	REPS	SETS	REST
SUPERSET # 1				
Glutes and Quads: One-Legged Squat with Ball	56	10–12	4	0 seconds
Hamstrings: Lying Hamstring Curl on Machine	100	10–12	4	60 seconds
Glutes and Quads: Ball Lunge	58	10–12	4	0 seconds
Hamstrings: Curl On All Fours	98	10–12	4	60 seconds
SUPERSET # 2				
Outer Thighs: Cable Leg Raise for Outer Thigh	86	10–12	4	0 seconds
Inner Thighs: Cable Leg Raise	78	10–12	4	60 seconds
Calves: Multi–Directional Calf Raises	118	10–12	4	0 seconds
Calves: Calf Press on Leg Press on Machine	110	10–12	4	60 seconds
AB WORKOUT				
Crunch on the Ball	122	20	2	15 seconds
Reverse Crunch with Legs Extended	124	20	2	15 seconds
Twist on the Ball	126	20	2	15 seconds
Jackknife on the Ball	128	20	2	15 seconds
Reverse Crunch	132	20	2	15 seconds
Plank with Rotation	130	20	2	15 seconds
Lower Back Extension	136	20	2	15 seconds

Cardio: Follow with 30 minutes of cardiovascular exercise such as elliptical, stationary bike, treadmill, or any other activity that will raise your heart rate to at least (220 – (Your Age)) x 0.75 +/– 10 beats.

DAY 5 — FRIDAY

EXERCISE	PAGE NO.	REPS	SETS	REST
SUPERSET # 1				
Glutes and Quads: Leg Press on Machine	62	10–12	4	0 seconds
Hamstrings: Hamstring Curl on the Ball	102	10–12	4	60 seconds
Glutes and Quads: One–Legged Butt Press with Ball	61	10–12	4	0 seconds
Hamstrings: Curl On All Fours	98	10–12	4	60 seconds
SUPERSET # 2				
Outer Thighs: Squat with Abduction	90	10–12	4	0 seconds
Inner Thighs: Lateral Lunge	72	10–12	4	60 seconds
Outer Thighs: Side Leg Kick	88	10–12	4	0 seconds
Inner Thighs: Wide Stance Squat	80	10–12	4	60 seconds
AB WORKOUT				
Crunch on the Ball	122	20	2	15 seconds
Reverse Crunch with Legs Extended	124	20	2	15 seconds
Twist on the Ball	126	20	2	15 seconds
Jackknife on the Ball	128	20	2	15 seconds
Reverse Crunch	132	20	2	15 seconds
Plank with Rotation	130	20	2	15 seconds
Lower Back Extension	136	20	2	15 seconds

Cardio: Follow with 30 minutes of cardiovascular exercise such as elliptical, stationary bike, treadmill, or any other activity that will raise your heart rate to at least (220 – (Your Age)) x 0.75 +/– 10 beats.

WEEKS 5 & 6

SPECIAL INSTRUCTIONS: Perform four sets of 8 to 10 repetitions for each exercise. Perform the exercises as giant sets as prescribed below.

DAY 1				MONDAY
EXERCISE	**PAGE NO.**	**REPS**	**SETS**	**REST**
GIANT SET # 1				
Glutes and Quads: Dumbbell Squat	48	8–10	4	0 seconds
Hamstrings: Hamstring Curl on the Ball	102	8–10	4	0 seconds
Glutes and Quads: Multi–Directional Lunges	50	8–10	4	0 seconds
Hamstrings: Deadlift	108	8–10	4	60 seconds
GIANT SET # 2				
Outer Thighs: Ball Abduction	94	8–10	4	0 seconds
Inner Thighs: Lateral Lunge onto BOSU or Step	74	8–10	4	0 seconds
Outer Thighs: Abductor on Machine	92	8–10	4	0 seconds
Inner Thighs: Adductor on Machine	76	8–10	4	60 seconds
AB WORKOUT				
Crunch on the Ball	122	20	3	15 seconds
Reverse Crunch with Legs Extended	124	20	3	15 seconds
Twist on the Ball	126	20	3	15 seconds
Jackknife on the Ball	128	20	3	15 seconds
Reverse Crunch	132	20	3	15 seconds
Plank with Rotation	130	20	3	15 seconds
Lower Back Extension	136	20	3	15 seconds

Cardio: Follow with 40 minutes of cardiovascular exercise such as elliptical, stationary bike, treadmill, or any other activity that will raise your heart rate to at least (220 – (Your Age)) x 0.75 +/– 10 beats.

DAYS 2, 4, AND 6 — TUESDAY, THURSDAY, AND SATURDAY

On Tuesdays, Thursdays, and Saturdays you can perform an upper body workout portion from the Advanced 14–Day Body Sculpting Program such as the one presented in *The Body Sculpting Bible for Women* followed by 40 minutes of cardiovascular exercise such as elliptical, stationary bike, treadmill, or any other activity that will raise your heart rate to at least (220 – (Your Age)) x 0.75 +/– 10 beats. For your upper body training, just follow the same repetition and rest schemes as the ones used for your lower-body workouts even if using the Advanced Workout from the original *Body Sculpting Bible*.

DAY 3 — WEDNESDAY

EXERCISE	PAGE NO.	REPS	SETS	REST
GIANT SET # 1				
Glutes and Quads: One–Legged Squat with Ball	56	8–10	4	0 seconds
Hamstrings: Lying Hamstring Curl on Machine	100	8–10	4	0 seconds
Glutes and Quads: Ball Lunge	58	8–10	4	0 seconds
Hamstrings: Curl On All Fours	98	8–10	4	60 seconds
GIANT SET # 2				
Outer Thighs: Cable Leg Raise for Outer Thigh	86	8–10	4	0 seconds
Inner Thighs: Cable Leg Raise	78	8–10	4	0 seconds
Calves: Multi–Directional Calf Raises	118	8–10	4	0 seconds
Calves: Calf Press on Leg Press Machine	110	8–10	4	60 seconds
AB WORKOUT				
Crunch on the Ball	122	20	3	15 seconds
Reverse Crunch with Legs Extended	124	20	3	15 seconds
Twist on the Ball	126	20	3	15 seconds
Jackknife on the Ball	128	20	3	15 seconds
Reverse Crunch	132	20	3	15 seconds
Plank with Rotation	130	20	3	15 seconds
Lower Back Extension	136	20	3	15 seconds

Cardio: Follow with 40 minutes of cardiovascular exercise such as elliptical, stationary bike, treadmill, or any other activity that will raise your heart rate to at least (220 – (Your Age)) x 0.75 +/– 10 beats.

DAY 5 — FRIDAY

EXERCISE	PAGE NO.	REPS	SETS	REST
GIANT SET # 1				
Glutes and Quads: Leg Press on Machine	62	8–10	4	0 seconds
Hamstrings: Hamstring Curl on the Ball	102	8–10	4	0 seconds
Glutes and Quads: One–Legged Butt Press with Ball	60	8–10	4	0 seconds
Hamstrings: Curl On All Fours	98	8–10	4	60 seconds
GIANT SET # 2				
Outer Thighs: Squat with Abduction	90	8–10	4	0 seconds
Inner Thighs: Lateral Lunge	72	8–10	4	0 seconds
Outer Thighs: Side Leg Kick	88	8–10	4	0 seconds
Inner Thighs: Wide Stance Squat	80	8–10	4	60 seconds
AB WORKOUT				
Crunch on the Ball	122	20	3	15 seconds
Reverse Crunch with Legs Extended	124	20	3	15 seconds
Twist on the Ball	126	20	3	15 seconds
Jackknife on the Ball	128	20	3	15 seconds
Reverse Crunch	132	20	3	15 seconds
Plank with Rotation	130	20	3	15 seconds
Lower Back Extension	136	20	3	15 seconds

Cardio: Follow with 40 minutes of cardiovascular exercise such as elliptical, stationary bike, treadmill, or any other activity that will raise your heart rate to at least (220 – (Your Age)) x 0.75 +/– 10 beats.

Appendix A
Daily Workout Journal

Use the log on the following page to keep track of your progress in your workouts.

A

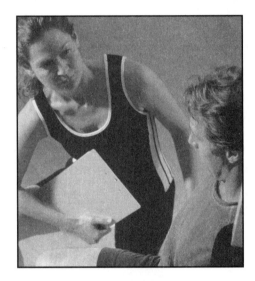

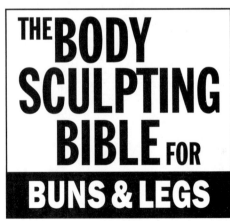

Daily Workout Journal   Week ⚪   Day ⚪

	Exercise	Rest	Set 1		Set 2		Set 3		Set 4	
	Main (Alternate)		Reps	Weight	Reps	Weight	Reps	Weight	Reps	Weight
Superset or Giant Set 1										
Superset or Giant Set 2										
Superset or Giant Set 3										
Superset or Giant Set 4										
Abs										

Cardio

Cardio Activity: Notes:

Average Heart Rate:

Duration:

Use the Daily Workout Journal to keep track of your workout. Photocopy this page as many times as you need.

Appendix B
Daily Nutrition Journal

Good nutrition boils down to some simple basics:

Always try to use natural foods. Avoid using canned or prepared foods as they usually contain too much fat, sodium, and carbs.

Stay within plus or minus 10 grams of the recommended amount of carbs and proteins, plus or minus 5 grams for fats.

Always choose low-fat protein sources. Don't worry about incurring a fat deficiency since the supplements program takes care of the need for essential fatty acids. Besides, there are trace amounts of fats even in low-fat protein sources.

If you choose to include skim milk in your diet, remember that it not only has protein but also simple carbs. Therefore, count milk as both. Since the carbs in milk are simple carbs, this should be used only in the post-workout meal. However, if your schedule requires you to include more protein shakes throughout the day, and you will rely on the carbs in skim milk, add a teaspoon of flaxseed oil to the milk to slow down the release of simple carbs into the bloodstream.

Try to include fibrous carbs in at least two meals.

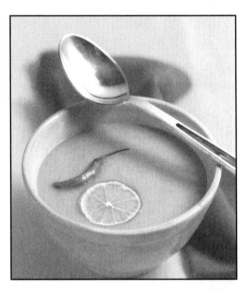

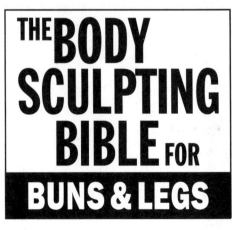

Daily Nutrition Journal Week ◯ Day ◯

	Food	Serving Size	Calories	Carbs (grams)	Protein (grams)	Fat (grams)	
Meal 1							Meal 1
Meal 2							Meal 2
Meal 3							Meal 3
Meal 4							Meal 4
Meal 5							Meal 5
Meal 6							Meal 6
	TOTAL						

Use the Daily Nutrition Journal to keep track of your diet. Photocopy the page as many times as you need.

Appendix C
Useful Resources

WWW.BODYSCULPTINGBIBLE.COM

A powerful resource for anyone seeking advice, knowledge, and more. Loaded with news, fitness tips, and discussion forums, this is a must-see.

WWW.HRFIT.NET

A visit here will reward you with a well-rounded bushel of information written by Hugo Rivera, ranging from how to design a workout routine to how to select or reject a food supplement.

WWW.JVFITNESS.COM

This site is owned by James Villepigue, featured Fitness Trainer of *Live with Regis and Kelly*. A visit to this site will provide you with information on weight training, nutrition, supplementation, and kid/teenage training.

WWW.LOSEFATANDGAINMUSCLE.COM

For information on bodybuilding training, mass building tactics, and nutrition, this renowned site offers no-holds barred information, and brings you into the trenches of the real-deal bodybuilding lifestyle.

WWW.BODYTECHONLINE.COM

The home of bodybuilding coach and fitness guru Tim Gardner who owns Body* Tech Fitness Emporium, a fine 12,000 sq. ft health and fitness club in the Florida Tampa Bay area.

WWW.BODYBUILDING.COM

Tons of free information on anything you need to know about bodybuilding and fitness, written by several experts in the industry. They also carry most supplement brands in the market selling them at a huge discount.

WWW.BODYBUILDING.ABOUT.COM

Free articles on training, nutrition, supplementation and recuperation written by Hugo Rivera, James Villepigue, and other top industry experts.

WWW.IRONMASTER.COM

Home of the Quick-Lock Dumbbells, where you will find very economical, sturdy, and safe pieces of fitness equipment.

WWW.POWERBLOCKS.COM

A good resource for home fitness equipment.

WWW.FITNESSFACTORY.COM

Great place to fulfill your home gym equipment needs.

WWW.PROLAB.COM

Prolab is one of the top notch companies in the industry that carries all of the basic supplements that bodybuilders need at very affordable prices.

WWW.DAVEDRAPER.COM

Dave is a bodybuilding legend, winner of the Mr. America, Mr. World, and Mr. Universe titles. In his site, Dave shares his extensive knowledge in a very straight-forward, simple, and almost poetic manner.

WWW.MUSCLEBUILDINGDIET.COM

Owned by Todd Mendelsohn, a former Mr. Central Florida who works as a nutrition/training consultant. If you want more advanced tailor made programs for bulking up then this is the place to go.